Praise for

"*Incredibly practical and uplifting, this book shows simple and proven ways out of an unhealthy, stressful lifestyle—from what you eat, how you exercise, and what you think and feel to a balanced life abounding with joy, vitality, and sacredness. The Joy Factor will have a major impact on your life.*"
—JOHN ROBBINS, AUTHOR OF *Diet for a New America*

"The Joy Factor *contains all of the essential ingredients to live our very best lives—physically, mentally, emotionally, and spiritually. Susan has a gift for taking complex research, scientific studies, and personal experiences and distilling them down to the most essential, empowering, and practical level. I especially appreciate her personal stories and how she brings insight to life lessons we all need to learn in order to live our highest potential. Susan's book will enrich your experience of living, too!*"
—VICTORIA MORAN, AUTHOR OF *Creating a Charmed Life*

"The Joy Factor *is an exquisitely beautiful book, with profound depth, sound health advice, and practical application techniques that will touch your heart and transform your life forever. Sensational!*"
—ELLEN TART-JENSEN, PhD, AUTHOR OF *Health Is Your Birthright*

"*The perfect blend of modern research and ageless wisdom. Susan Smith Jones's sound and practical guidance, along with the inspiring personal stories about her life and work with her clients, will help everyone awaken to a new understanding of what living fully, celebrating life, and creating vibrant health are all about. The Joy Factor will touch your heart and change your life for the better.*"
—ALEXANDRA STODDARD, AUTHOR OF *You Are Your Choices: 50 Ways to Live the Good Life*

"*This combination book/workbook is sure to be a welcome companion for anyone seeking to bring vitality and radiant health into their lives. Whether you are 18 or 88, consider this required reading for bringing peace and high-level wellness to your life. I wholeheartedly recommend it to everyone!*"
—NEAL BARNARD, MD, FOUNDER AND PRESIDENT, PHYSICIANS COMMITTEE FOR RESPONSIBLE MEDICINE; AUTHOR OF *Breaking the Food Seduction*

"*What an absolute joy to read. This thought-provoking, beautifully written, and empowering book breaks through the barriers of conventional health, healing, and medicine and presents an innovative and highly effective program for creating radiant health, youthful vitality, and a balanced life.*"
—Rebecca Linder Hintze, author of *Healing Your Family History*

"*I always look forward to Susan's books, and this one was well worth the wait.* The Joy Factor *inspires and empowers the reader to 'seize the day' while providing a well-conceived blueprint for creating a life filled with health, happiness, joy, and peace. A superb book.*"
—Gabriel Cousens, MD, author of *There Is a Cure for Diabetes*

"*For more than thirty years, Dr. Susan Smith Jones has been living and teaching the material presented in* The Joy Factor. *She has superbly distilled the most essential issues and created a beautifully-written guide that's easy to understand and, more importantly, easy to apply in our lives. Once I started reading, I could hardly put it down. Read this life-changing, sagacious book.*"
—Dianne Warren, author of *Vegetable Soup/The Fruit Bowl*

"*What a magnificent book! Be sure to check out the workbook at the back, which invites us to look within ourselves to examine and understand more fully our beliefs, attitudes, heart-feelings, needs, desires, and our highest vision for ourselves and the world. This section made a profound difference in my life and will doubtless change your life for the better, too. I am recommending it to all of my friends, family, and on my radio shows.*"
—Nick Lawrence, radio/tv talk show host and personality

"*You will want to add this glorious, delightful book to your home library, keep it front and center, and refer to it often. You will thank your lucky stars that you have this book as your guide to creating optimal wellness, living fully, and celebrating life. Keep several copies on hand, because you will want to give them as gifts. Kudos to Susan!*"
—Anita Finley, radio talk show host and publisher of *Boomer Times*

The Joy factor

10 SACRED PRACTICES FOR RADIANT HEALTH

Also by Susan Smith Jones

The *Joy* *factor*

10 SACRED PRACTICES FOR RADIANT HEALTH

SUSAN SMITH JONES, PhD

CONARI
PRESS

First published in 2011 by Conari Press,
An imprint of Red Wheel/Weiser, LLC
With offices at:
500 Third Street, Suite 230
San Francisco, CA 94107
www.redwheelweiser.com

ISBN: 978-1-57324-478-7

Library of Congress Cataloging-in-Publication Data is available upon request.

Cover and text design by Linda Kosarin / TheArtDepartment.biz
Typeset in Granjon
Cover photograph © urbancow/iStockPhoto
Printed in the United States of America
TS
10 9 8 7 6 5 4 3 2 1
Text paper contains a minimum of 30% post-consumer-waste material.

This book is dedicated, in loving memory,

to my beautiful mother, June. Through her invincible courage,

resplendent spirit, and shining example,

she taught me how to love deeply,

live fully, follow my heart, practice kindness, offer compassion,

and celebrate life. She will always be my most positive role

model and the person I most want to mirror.

GRATITUDES

To my dear friend and executive editor at Red Wheel Weiser, Caroline Pincus: This book would not have been possible without your support and encouragement. You took my vision and dream and helped me turn it into a glorious writing experience from the beginning to the end. Your guidance is invaluable, and your loving friendship is immeasurable to me. You are one of my earth angels.

To the folks at Red Wheel Weiser: Jan Johnson, Michael Kerber, Bonni Hamilton, Greg Brandenburgh, Dennis Fitzgerald, Amber Guetebier, Susie Pitzen, Lisa Trudeau, Rachel Leach, Nicole Deneka, Martha Knauf, Jordan Overby, Jim Warner, Lauren Rouleau, Debbie Huffman, Angie Martinez, Hillary Peacock, Sylvia Hopkins, Judi O'Donnell, Colleen Doheny, Alex Huffman, and Devin Bebout. Everyone has been a joy to work with and always so supportive. Thank you for your help in making our book an international bestseller.

A special thanks also to Linda Kosarin for the cover and interior design.

To my friends and extended family who have supported me in this project from day one: Betty Wetzel, Bob Deskins, Ralph Rudser, Ginny Swabek, Junia Chambers, Jackie Benoit, Edwin Basye, Bonnie Ross, Helen Guppy, Colleen and Dave, Lisa Ray, and David Craddock. Your loving kindness, thoughtful conversation, and guidance throughout the process are deeply appreciated.

You'll notice that I write about my mother, June, and my grandmother, Fritzie. I am so blessed to have these positive role models guiding me to this day in all my work and throughout my life. "Follow your dreams," they always used to say to me, and this book is definitely a dream come true. Thank you.

CONTENTS

Chapter 1 Set the Bar High
I CHOOSE TO LIVE MY BEST LIFE *1*

If It's to Be, It's Up to Me • Your Reality Reflects Your Thoughts
and Intentions • Success Is an Inside Job • The Role of the Body
in Self-Mastery • Love Is the Main Ingredient • Divinity Is
Another Main Ingredient • Mary June's Transformation
• The Power of Commitment • Turn Adversity to Advantage
• Personal Commitment Statement • Make a Difference

Chapter 2 Act with Kindness
I CHOOSE TO SPREAD HAPPINESS WHEREVER I GO *27*

The Religion of Kindness • Let Your Heart-Light Shine
• Reach Out and Touch Someone • The Health Benefits of
Small Pleasures • The Health Benefits of Love and Kindness
• Showing Kindness Day to Day

Chapter 3 Celebrate the Child in You
I CHOOSE TO APPROACH LIFE AS A PLAYFUL ADVENTURE *45*

Childlike versus Childish • Let the Child in You Come Out
to Play • Be All That You Can Be • Give Fantasy Its Wings
and Fly • Living in the Present • Don't Be Afraid to Make
Mistakes or Fail • Accept the World as It Is
• Laugh and Be a Little Silly

Foreword

I have long subscribed to the idea that all of life is a choice. When we let ourselves ultimately come to believe in the power of being a "choice-making" human being, we begin to take total responsibility for our unique destinies and ourselves. Susan Jones provides us with a beautifully useful elaboration on this theme of choosing our own greatness in virtually all life areas. She has taken great pains to provide extremely valuable information on how to take total control of ourselves by first and foremost taking responsibility for the quality of the journey that we call life.

In simple, easy-to-read, and most importantly, easy-to-apply language, this book outlines an approach to living that is possible for every single reader to achieve if he or she is willing to make it happen for themselves. Regardless of your current state of physical or emotional disrepair, you can take this book, read carefully, and begin now to create vibrant health and bring serenity and sacred balance into your body and life.

A strong thread of spirituality and higher consciousness thinking is woven through the pages of *The Joy Factor*. Susan cannot help but write from this perspective, because I know her to be respectful of the divine forces operating ubiquitously in each and every one of us. Susan believes strongly in the importance of love in each of our lives. Not the kind of love that requires a partner in order to be fulfilled, but the divine love that is itself the harmony that holds every living cell together. Without internal harmony, a cell will attack and attempt to devour the cell adjacent to it and will ultimately destroy the entire organism. So it is with divine love. Each of us is a cell in the body called humanity. When we have harmony within, we cooperate with the cells next to us, and when this harmony or love is missing, we fight our adjacent cells, leading to destruction of the totality of all humanity. When we fight anything, we become weaker, for in so doing we are violating the very principle of harmony and cooperation that holds the universe together. You will see Susan's enormous regard for this spiritual (not necessarily religious, but spiritual) force that guides the universe and each life form that occupies its own unique place in this perfect universe.

Recent efforts by chemists and other scientists have produced a synthetic product that looks, tastes, smells, feels, and acts like wheat. To the naked eye it appears that this is definitely wheat. However, when it is placed in the ground, something quite strange happens that sets it apart from authentic wheat. It will not grow! Despite its appearance and nutritional make-up, synthetic wheat will not grow and reproduce naturally. What is missing? The absent ingredient is the Life Force that can never be reproduced synthetically.

So it is with each of us. We need the higher elements in order to grow, along with a life plan that incorporates authentic ingredients for choosing to be vibrantly healthy, happy, and fully alive. Susan sprinkles her writing with marvelous quotations from the masters, both historic and contemporary, who have all made their own unique contributions to the betterment of humankind. Her writing is concise and useful, and the subject matter is universal: improving the quality of life for all of us. *The Joy Factor* can help you forget about synthetic happiness, artificial health, and phony fulfillment and replace them with a genuine, life-enhancing formula that will help you not only feel better but also grow and flourish, just like real wheat does when placed in a natural setting.

Everything we experience is a choice. Our personalities are the result of the choices we make. Our level of fitness is the result of those same opportunities to choose to be healthy. Our emotional condition is a consequence of our choices. When you really consider this concept of choice, it boils down to the way that we choose to think. We become what we think about all day long. Thus, our personality, state of health, and emotional stability all revolve around thinking. Learn to think health and visualize yourself as a success, and eventually your actions will follow those internal self-pictures. It can be no other way. Our thinking is our mental practice. With enough practice you will achieve what you desire.

Susan's approach is to help you to see that you are important enough to seek your own full measure of happiness and success, and that you are divine enough, just by the nature of your existence, to be heard. As you read through the pages of this powerful book, remind yourself that you are indeed divine enough to be answered. Think of a puzzle with one piece missing and realize that the entire picture is incomplete without that one piece. Then see yourself as one piece in this entire picture called humanity and that the whole thing is incomplete without you. That is how important you are. Your completeness makes us all whole, and Susan's outstanding book will help you not only to grasp this notion but also to take action, beginning now, to correct any limits you may have placed on yourself.

—WAYNE W. DYER,
author of *Excuses Begone!* and *Change Your Thoughts, Change Your Life*

If you can dream it, you can do it.
—WALT DISNEY

Be the change you wish to see in the world.
—GANDHI

When I look into the future, it's so bright it burns my eyes.
—OPRAH WINFREY

Preface

There is a single magic, a single power, a single salvation, and a single happiness, and that is called loving.
—James Allen

People are always blaming their circumstances for what they are. I don't believe in circumstances. The people who get on in this world are the people who get up and look for the circumstances they want and if they can't find them, make them.
—George Bernard Shaw

For as long as I can remember, I have enjoyed writing. Through writing, I have come to understand my life with more clarity, and to appreciate the lessons that have been sent my way. Over the years my life and my experience of being in this world have changed, just as I'm sure yours have. Expressing my thoughts and feelings on paper has frequently given me clues to how I might take care of unfinished business or unresolved conflict, and how I might identify the nugatory and troubling beliefs that keep me from being all I was created to be.

Before we continue on, there's something I think you should know about me. I've always had a penchant for words, so much so that I have a dictionary in every room of my home. If I were stranded on a desert island and could only take one book, it would be my dictionary, without a doubt. In fact, whenever I read a book—and I strive to read two to three books weekly—it only makes it to my list of favorites if it teaches me at least twelve new words.

Through the reading process, I keep a dictionary nearby, and I often write the meaning of a new word, complete with its usage, derivation, and so on, right in the margin of the book. That way, if I'm ever re-reading the book and forget the meaning of the word, the definition is right there on the page.

As you'll discover as you read this book, I've found special places to use some of my favorite choice yet underused words. I hope you're willing to be stretched a little, too. Maybe you too will find yourself reading with a dictionary by your side and develop a penchant for looking up words that are new to you.

In all my books, I also try to communicate the love I have for life. In this one, I hope to share on a very personal level the lessons that have been most important to me. I see this as a voyage we'll take together, an adventure of hope, renewal, rejoicing, and making choices. Your active participation is important, because it's not what we read that makes the difference in our lives but rather how we apply the ideas to ourselves. I love what Henry David Thoreau said about the books he preferred to read:

Books, not which afford us a cowering enjoyment,

but in which each thought is of unusual daring;

such as an idle person cannot read, and a timid one would not

be entertained by, which even make us dangerous to existing

institutions—such I call good books.

My greatest hope is that reading and participating in this book will help you turn your life into a magnificent adventure. You do make a difference. There is no one like you in this entire world, no one with your talents, your eyes, your heart, your fingerprints, or your dreams. You are inimitable and have been given the puissance and potential to make your life, and this world, any way you want it to be. It doesn't matter where you've been, what you've done in the past, how many mistakes you've made, or how old you are. Right now, right this moment, you can begin to make different choices. You can choose to be all that you were created to be—vibrantly healthy, happy, centered and balanced, successful, and peaceful. You can feel totally alive, filled with enthusiasm for life, the way you felt when you were a small child. Aliveness! Fully alive and thriving! It's a choice and it's your divine right.

As we spend some time together through these pages, you will discover some of the ways I have chosen to live healthfully and what I think living fully and living a serene, sacred life is all about. You will find out that it's more than just feeling fine physically. It's a joy and radiance for living such that each day and each and every moment can be a celebration.

Of course, I didn't wake up one morning and find that my life had simply turned around. The experience I refer to as my "wake-up call" is described in detail in my other books. Briefly, I fractured my back in an automobile accident, and the doctor told me I should be prepared for a life of pain, inactivity, and difficulty. The universe got my attention in a big way. That was many years ago, and although I didn't know how I would change my physical condition, I was determined to be well. With the help of wonderful teachers, I recognized that the Higher Power within me—the source of light and beauty that Robert Browning called "the imprisoned splendor"—had the answers and the ability to heal. I made a deep commitment to let go, live from inner guidance, and accept only vibrant health.

I am often asked about the people from whom I've learned the most, the ones who have had the most profound, positive influence on my life. There are eight. Jesus (my constant daily companion), Paramahansa Yogananda, and White Eagle are great spiritual teachers who have shown me the importance of practicing love and forgiveness and of living as a spiritual being in human form. I turn to their words often for inspiration.

Millions of people, me included, are inspired by Louise L. Hay. If you are one of those few who haven't read any of her 25 bestselling books, you may want to get a copy of her book, *Experience Your Good Now: Learning to Use Affirmations*. This reader-friendly gem will touch your heart, lift your spirit, and give you hope that anything and everything is possible, with enough faith, belief, and positive intention.

My glorious mom, June, was always a radiant example of joy, enthusiasm, perseverance, and love for everything and everyone. Her mettle was sustained by a heart of gold, and she instilled in me the values of high thinking, living my vision, never giving up, and following my heart. She was a wonderful blessing in my life. My grandmother, Fritzie, belongs on the list, too. She was peaceful, happy, independent, and self-reliant. She traveled the world, ate healthy foods, and led a simple life. Her example and loving words helped orchestrate my life, and I still feel her presence often. She also introduced me to the Essene.

As I write in chapter 7, my interest in the Essene began almost forty years ago when Fritzie taught me about this extraordinary community of people who lived from the second century BC to the first century AD. Jesus and His family were associated with the Essene community. The Essenes were evolved people who had broken away from the mainstream of Jewish thought several hundred years before the time of Jesus. They were the spiritual heroes of their day, basing their whole lives on spiritual development and achievement. They were devout lovers of peace, and were particularly orderly and clean in their habits. Most important, they were a people who believed in action—in doing rather than talking and practicing themselves what they then taught to others. They actually lived their philosophy of nonresistance, harmlessness, returning good for evil, and above all, blending the individual spirit with the Spirit of Infinite Love, much the way Fritzie and Peace Pilgrim (mentioned below) lived.

The Essene lifestyle required a discipline and purity of body, mind, and spirit that went beyond the practice of the typical religious person of that time. The Essenes developed self-sufficient communities in a remote desert area in order to make it easier for them to focus on God. As part of their teaching of compassion and love for all life, the Essenes taught vegetarianism. They were said to eat primarily live, or raw, foods and were reported by anthropological historians to live an average of 120 years.

Finally, there's Peace Pilgrim, a great source of inspiration for me, a walking, breathing example of living peacefully. In fact, Fritzie reminded me of Peace Pilgrim in many ways. For close to thirty years she traveled all over North America—all fifty states, the ten provinces of Canada, and parts of Mexico—sharing her thoughts about peace. She went on foot, never asking for anything and without one penny in her pocket. All she had were the clothes she wore and the sustenance she received along the way. Her motto was as simple as her life: "This is the way of peace: overcome evil with good, and falsehood with truth, and hatred with love." Only one thing could inspire such a long journey and provide her with the strength to see it through, and that was faith—absolute, uncompromising faith in herself and in God. On peace, she said, "When you find peace within yourself, you become the kind of person who can live at peace with others."

During the months following my accident, and to this day, I have continued to make changes in my lifestyle, behavior, thoughts, and attitudes. I've learned to bring more consciousness to my living, to pay attention to life and to observe its patterns, using the ones that support me in new ways and changing the ones that don't. I now choose to live more deeply, to find the intention beneath my intention, and always to talk things over with God before making any decisions. There is so much more to health than a strong body and a clear mind. Being vibrantly healthy and serene implies a harmonious balance of one's physical, emotional, mental, and spiritual self—and a recognition that these are not separate. We are whole beings created in the image and likeness of God.

Next to the word God you'll see that I placed an asterisk. I know many people who have trouble with that word. If you're one of them, consider any of these synonyms or create the word or words that feel the best to you. In the pages of this book, I'll switch between words that resonate most strongly in my heart.

Love

Light	The Infinite
Lord	Allah
Heavenly Father	The Force
Divine Mother	Tao
Peace	Life Force
Higher Power	Universal Energy or Force
Divinity	Life
Creator	The Divine
Spirit	Heart Light

You'll discover that I often refer to the spiritual side of life, the sacred, and God. Let me take a few moments to clarify what these words mean to me. My concept of God is the essence of life— Love—the universal force that both surrounds us and is within us and which connects us all to one another. Thoreau expressed it well when he said, "Our religion is where our love is." For me, spirituality is more than performance of sacraments, rituals, and songs. I express the spirit within me by the way I live, by my belief and faith in a Creator, by my reverence for nature, and by my desire to nurture humankind. I am deeply in love with all people, all creation, and with life itself. Life is sacred, and every step we take is on holy ground. We must bring sacredness into all of our daily activities, which include our thoughts, words, and actions. This is why the chapters of this book are structured around the word "sacredness."

I suggest that you read the book through once in its entirety. Then read it again, slowly and deliberately, reading no more than one chapter a day. Think about the topic for a day. Absorb it. Practice living it, if you feel called to do so, and make sure you participate in the Self-Discovery Questions and Action Choices in the Appendix. Think of what I've said about writing, and don't pass over this "workbook." Take time with each item. No one has to see what you've written. It should be your private, personal transformation journal. This special section will assist you in getting to know yourself better. And after all, isn't that the key to living our highest potential?

My automobile accident taught me that dark nights of the soul can reveal the true purpose of suffering: that out of our pain we can rise, expand, grow, conquer, and achieve new and ever-better things. Like the butterfly that is strengthened by its desperate struggle to break out of a constricting cocoon, we too can emerge stronger, wiser, and more resilient because of the painful, difficult times in our lives. In those times we learn to simplify life, clarify values, sort out priorities, and cherish our true friends.

I like to think that even without a catastrophic wake-up call, I would have discovered the tremendous power of commitment, belief, and faith. Faith is the certainty of an inner knowing, appearances notwithstanding. Commitment links me, both mind and heart, to aspirations, goals, and people. When I believe in a relationship, a plan, or a task, and give myself wholeheartedly to it, I do well. When I am God-centered, however, I do my best. I bring love and compassion to every interaction with others, and inspiration to every activity I undertake.

What I have found happening in my life is that, as I gradually develop a quieter and clearer awareness of the Higher Power in me, my living habits naturally come into harmony with my total environment, with my past involvements, present interests, and future priorities. When we are in touch with our innermost Self, when we begin to discover who we truly are, and when we choose to commit to live from inner guidance, rather than play the victims of the world we see, the changes in our lives come about naturally. It was Emily Dickinson who said "I dwell in possibility." We all have unlimited possibility to create the life of our highest dreams. I know you can do it.

To laugh often and much; to win the respect of intelligent people and the affection of children; to earn the appreciation of honest critics and endure the betrayal of false friends; to appreciate beauty; to find the best in others; to leave the world a bit better, whether by a healthy child, a garden patch, or a redeemed social condition; to know even one life has breathed easier because you have lived. This is to have succeeded.
—Ralph Waldo Emerson

My life belongs to the whole community, and as long as I live, it is my privilege to do for it whatsoever I can. I want to be thoroughly used up when I die, for the harder I work, the more I live. I rejoice in life for its own sake. Life is no "brief candle" to me. It is a sort of splendid torch, which I have got hold of for the moment, and I want to make it burn as brightly as possible before handing it on to future generations.
—George Bernard Shaw

Resplendent Living

We are one, after all, you and I, together we suffer, together exist.
And forever we recreate each other.
—TEILHARD DE CHARDIN

Of all the beautiful truths pertaining to the soul which have been restored
and brought to life in this age, none is more gladdening or fruitful of divine
promise and confidence than this—that man is the master of thought, the
molder of character, and the maker and shaper of condition, environment,
and destiny.
—JAMES ALLEN

As I travel the country and the world giving motivational talks, whether in person or during radio and television talk shows, I meet countless people who all seem to be experiencing the same thing—what I refer to as a "busyness" or "hurry sickness." Everyone seems to be rushing around—from the moment they wake up until they go to bed at night—and it just seems to be getting worse. I read an article recently in *The New York Times* disclosing that one-third of all Americans are always in a state of rush. Where are we all going?

In one of my all-time favorite books, *The Little Prince* by Saint Exupéry (yes, I also read it in French and had to consult my trusty English/French dictionary companion several times on each page), there's a section in which the little prince is in the railway station. He asks where all the people walking back and forth all over the place are going. Someone replies, "Even the engineer doesn't know where he's going." Can you relate to this in your life, too?

When you reach the end of your life, I guarantee you that you will not be wishing you had led a more stressful, harried existence and that you spent more time rushing around. My grandmother, Fritzie, was always right: she often reminded me that it's the simple pleasures that make life worth living—being with your friends; laughing much and often; celebrating the sunrise and sunset; enjoying your children, grandchildren, and pets; carving out time to stroll in Nature and appreciate its bounty, and so on— these are what bring sweetness and pure joy to living. These are the things that you'll remember with great fondness and that will bring a smile to your face. This is what living a sacred life is all about. We all need to create space in our days to experience the true sacredness of life and feel the joy of living fully.

Ask yourself the following questions:

- Am I feeling physically, emotionally, and spiritually off-kilter?
- Have I lost some joy of living?
- Do I feel overwhelmed by life and too much daily stress?
- Or, perhaps, have I ever experienced, or do I wish to experience, the true sacredness of life?

Because you are reading this book, I have a feeling that you've answered "yes" to many of these questions. Well, you've come to the right place, because my goal in this book is to gently and lovingly guide you back to your true nature—your sacred heart center where each day and each moment can be worth celebrating—even in the midst of stress and chaos. The door to your sacred center, which by now might be rusted shut for lack of use, is simply waiting for you to open it. All it takes is your willingness to turn the knob and enter, surrendering to the gifts and miracles waiting for you. These gifts and miracles are already inside you, where they have always been. This sacred center is within you.

Accessing it is not, it should be noted, something you do just once, say on January first, when you're all psyched up and motivated to make personal changes. It's a process you can choose to engage each and every day, preferably early every morning as you greet the day.

Living a sacred life involves a blending of body, mind, and spirit. Remember, the body reflects the mind, and the mind reflects the spirit. It doesn't matter whether you start with the body by choosing to upgrade your diet or exercise daily, or with your mind by choosing to think more positively, or if you simply focus on Spirit and add in some special prayer or meditation time each day. All of these endeavors will lead to the same place—your sacred center—and a life rich in joy, vibrant health, and soul-satisfaction. Prayer, as I see it, is the way we reconnect with our sacred essence, and this oneness with the Divine is our lifeline to endless inspiration and vitality.

Hummingbirds are some of my favorite teachers, shining examples of how to live a sacred life. In a Papyrus card store, I read how legends say that hummingbirds float free of time, carrying our hopes for love, joy, and celebration. The hummingbird's delicate grace reminds us that life is rich, beauty is everywhere, every personal connection has meaning, and that laughter is life's sweetest creation. So my hope for all of us is that we become like hummingbirds, savoring each moment as it passes, embracing all that life has to offer, and celebrating the joy of everyday. That's true sacredness.

If you have already perused the table of contents, you will see that the chapter titles in this book flow from the acronym SACREDNESS. Think of each of these letters (and chapters) as windows lighting the way to your sacred center. With each chapter, your understanding of how to live fully and bring a sacred balance back into your body and life will grow. This moment can be a fresh start for you—a new beginning and a whole new way to create your very best life.

Let's start fresh right now. If you are willing to move forward and embrace a new way of living, then let's begin this journey together. I will be with you every step of the way, holding your hand and giving you encouragement.

Right now you have the power and ability to transform and enrich the quality of your life and life on this planet. You can be all you were meant to be. No one has ever stopped you but you. Yes, you can live a luminous, munificent life, glowing with self-esteem and verve and radiating strength. But you must make a conscious choice to do so. This moment—right now—can be a new beginning. No longer do you need to repeat the past, worry about the future, or struggle through life as a victim of circumstance. If you begin to live today—absorbed in the present moment, letting your Heart-Light shine, being responsible and accountable for who you are and what you want to become—you will begin to experience every day a life more splendid, more wondrous, and more magical than you ever dreamed possible.

Taking responsibility is the first step, as is knowing that the responsibility is squarely on your shoulders. You cannot blame something or someone outside yourself for your own failure to live your vision. It's simply a matter of creating what you want.

It isn't easy to accept that you have the power to choose, because you have probably been taught, as I was, to seek answers outside yourself. We can all learn something from outside sources, whatever they are, but the true teachers teach us to look within. The answers to the really important questions, the spiritual ones, can be found only by turning inward. Life and Love dwell within each of us. If we really look, we find that we are never alone. We also find that we are the gift and miracle we've been seeking, and when we start to live fully, we inspire excellence in all who touch and share our lives.

We must start by remembering that we have a body. We take good care of our body by feeding it healthy foods and exercising regularly. We also have a mind, and most of us nurture that by thinking, reading, writing, and communicating with others. But we are a soul above all, and if we don't shepherd the soul by bringing sacredness and balance into our body and life, we won't be complete.

In this new century and millennium, I believe that the individuals who will thrive are not necessarily those with the most accolades, achievements, or material possessions. Having a cell phone, a high-speed computer, a GPS, and a smartphone might make you feel plugged into the world of the future, but the only thing you might really be is wired. It's the people who are *internally* plugged in, the people who are deeply connected to their inner sacredness and spirituality, who will thrive and be champions in the 21st century. Of this I am sure.

The way to heal disharmony in your life and body and to reconnect with your sacred nature is to realize that, first and foremost, you are a spiritual being. Vibrant health and healing stem in large part from embracing your inner self: from the mental caress of meditation, prayer rich with belief, the soulful stirrings of human touch, knowing you are unconditionally loved by the Divine Light within you, and the resolution of conflict, anger, resentment, and hopelessness. Your Higher Power is like your soul's pilot light: it can choke in the face of deadlines, stress, traffic, days scheduled minute by minute, not telling the truth, not honoring your feelings, and not following your heart. You must choose to take ownership of your own soul and become the master of your life by harnessing the sacred within you and bringing it into everything you do and create.

I believe that all endeavors toward attaining better health are feckless unless the healthy body is seen and used as a temple in which Spirit dwells. Because of my belief, my emphasis is on

- physical exercise
- proper diet

- high thinking
- simple living

As mentioned previously, the body reflects the mind, and the mind reflects the spirit—hence the motivation to attain better health. Thoreau once said, "How prompt we are to satisfy the hunger and thirst of our bodies; how slow to satisfy the hunger and thirst of our souls." If we want to nourish both, we see the body not as a lump of flesh but rather as a noble instrument; within it is the source of all power. All we have to do is tap into it. Wisdom, Light, and Love are within each of us and make up the ribbon that unites us all together.

Life teaches us how to live. I am often asked if today's busy world can put one's spirituality at risk. Yes, it's easy to get caught up in the intense pace and stress of today's hectic lifestyle, especially if we've forgotten the truth of our being. The Life Force within us is diminished by misguided or pernicious attitudes about pain and growth, by our limiting beliefs and destructive self-definitions, and by judging others far more frequently than it is by disease or debacles. We have a tendency to approve or disapprove of others, and ourselves, according to superficial standards and labels of acceptability and achievement—when we should be learning to love. Finding the way to honor the sacredness within and around us heals and enriches life. We must come back to and embrace our authentic selves—this is sometimes a difficult thing to do.

Actually, we are all more than we know. Wholeness is never lost, it is only forgotten. We all need a strong foundation of practical spirituality based on the realization that we are co-creators with the ultimate source of power and creativity. We all have access to the universal creative power. We are tied directly to it. When we take our highest dreams seriously and focus on what we want, the natural pull of the universe will serve as a co-creative force that leads us to any goal we truly feel worthy to receive. With that type of partnership, I believe that anything is possible.

What I see happen with so many people is that they give up easily when their quest is challenged. I have found in my own life that stumbling blocks and challenges are just opportunities to learn and grow. Nothing keeps us from going ahead except our own thoughts and self-imposed limitations. We must stop vying with other people and judging from the appearances of so-called "reality" and have enough faith to choose a loftier perspective on life. Then we can move toward what we want by taking action. Each chapter of this book is devoted to a certain kind of life-enhancing action.

Through decades of research into Eastern philosophies and Western medicine, I've come to understand and appreciate how much the lines of demarcation between science and spirituality are diminishing. It is an irrefutable fact that we can't separate body, mind, and spirit. Science corroborates that when we live with a positive attitude—with faith, hope, and love in our hearts—we boost our immunity, have more energy, look younger, and stave off disease. Furthermore, scientists now agree that those people who meditate regularly not only handle stress better but look years younger than those who don't meditate. It's that simple. Especially in these times, we can't afford not to meditate.

For more than 35 years I have practiced meditation and studied the work of the venerable spiritual leader, Paramahansa Yogananda, founder of the Self-Realization Fellowship. Through his work, including the classic *Autobiography of a Yogi*, I have learned to see my life from a new perspective. The essence of his philosophy is that we need to live more in the presence of God and look inward for the answers in life. I have always had those beliefs on my own, but his books and lessons have reminded me in very practical terms that I can live a more spiritual life in a physical world and not get caught up in the frenzy of it all, especially not a frenzy of my own devising.

When Yogananda was alive, he always emphasized "plain living and high thinking," and that is how I choose to live. I want my life to radiate my devotion to God and my loving reverence and concern for all fellow beings, creatures, and life itself. Chapter 6 is devoted to meditation and other methods of expanding health and spiritual awareness.

I believe that Spirit speaks to us daily through our intuition and what we call "coincidences." Throughout our lives, coincidences lead us toward the attainment of our life's purpose. By increasing our awareness and remaining connected to our Source, we can see coincidences happening all around us when we ask the right questions. The answers are easy—it's the questions that are sometimes difficult. We must keep our energy at maximum level to be receptive to the messages that come to us through intuitive thoughts, daydreams, night dreams, and especially from people who show up on our path. And we must consciously develop our intuition.

Intuition is knowing something without thinking about it. I believe it's the voice of God within us. Too often we run away from ourselves, filling our lives with constant activity. We don't take time to be still, forget outside activities, and quell mental chattering. But intuition can be nurtured in a variety of ways, which I also describe in chapter 6. The more you act on your intuitive hunches, the stronger and more readily available they become. As you grow more sensitive to your oneness with God and life, you will become more intuitive. Receiving inner messages clearly comes when you learn to give up the analyzing, reasoning, doubting, and limiting part of your mind. The best way to strengthen intuitive power is just to sit still and listen. Turn within and pay attention.

If you don't like your current circumstances—if you want to lose weight, tone up your body, have more energy, live a more prosperous, peaceful life, and create vibrant health—you can do it. When you invite and allow Love (God, Heavenly Father, Divine Mother, Life Force, Light, Divinity, Lord, Source, Creator) to be the guiding force in your life, you become empowered, and this connection to your inner power creates miracles in your body and life and the lives of others. And changes that are loved into being are permanent.

Once we discover the sacred connection to our Source, we come to realize that we are all magnificent spiritual beings having a human experience here on spaceship Earth. We can choose to see this glorious universe as alive and mysterious, ultimately benevolent and orderly. Intention, consciousness, discovery, and synchronicity are magical and all around us. Every day the world presents us with miracles waiting for our awareness. Life-giving colorful fruits and vegetables are miracles. So are hummingbirds, butterflies, horses, sunsets and sunrises, shooting stars, the fragrance of roses, puppies and kittens, and our remarkable bodies that house the loving spirit within. Hidden beneath the wrapping of every experience is a new opportunity to know the joy and wonder of love.

One of the most important lessons I've learned is that if I'm facing a challenge—whether it's pertaining to health, relationships, finances, or whatever—all I need to do is turn my focus from the challenge to God and let the Divinity reveal the hidden gift within it. We're given the circumstances we require for our awakening.

Loving all aspects of your life, regardless of the challenges that inevitably come along, opens doors and lets in light, energy, and joy. Love yourself out of sheer gratitude for existence. Love the mystery of life and the process of creating what you want. Paramahansa Yogananda said, "Droplets of love sparkle in true souls, but in Spirit alone is found the sea of love." When you love, you become transformed spiritually. To quote *A Course in Miracles*, "Every loving thought is true. Everything else is an appeal for healing and help, regardless of the form it takes."

The more you love, the more you come to realize you don't need to force things. Jesus' teachings emphasize the importance of living from the love that is always within each of us. The *Tao-Te-Ching*, the classic Chinese manual on the art of living known in English as *The Book of the Way*, was written by the sage Lao-Tzu, whose large-heartedness, humor, and wisdom grace every page. He teaches that the true way is "to do by not doing," a paradigm for non-action, the purest and most effective form of action. He wrote, "The way to do is to be." For a long time, this has been one of my favorite maxims. You don't need to force things. Let go and let God. Or, as the Buddha put it at the end of his long life, "Be a light unto yourself."

The Joy Factor offers practical ways of living a serene, sacred, and balanced life and makes being vibrantly healthy, strong, and fit an achievable goal. This is how I've done my best to live for thirty-five years, and I know this way of living works. Of course I haven't always been a paragon, but every time I've fallen off my path, I've learned valuable lessons that I share in my books and workshops and with clients. We can all learn from one another. I've taught my holistic program to thousands of people around the country, and I receive countless letters each year highlighting their positive results.

It all begins with getting back to the basics—things our grandmothers probably told us that we didn't really want to hear about back then. Simple things like eating more fresh fruits and vegetables, including lots of greens (chapter 7), spending more time outdoors in nature (chapter 5), being more positive (chapter 8), giving joyfully to others (chapter 2), showing gratitude and trust (chapter 3), carving out times of solitude (chapter 9), and having faith in Love and God (every chapter).

If you're still not convinced that the journey to vibrant health is simple, because every day is already overflowing with activities, no matter how pedestrian, and there simply isn't time to start, I have a response for you. It is something I always tell people in my workshops, too. The time you feel least like starting something is precisely the time to forge ahead. Just the physical act of beginning will create the momentum and energy that will allow you to develop beyond your fear and toward your greatest accomplishments. Every step you take is on sacred ground. Everything about your life is sacred. The path to the sacred is your own body, heart, and mind, the history of your life, and the relationships and circumstances closest to you. Don't place limitations on your dreams or your Creator by doubting that you can reach your soul's desire and live a sacred life. If not here, where else can we engender joy, compassion, and happiness?

When we choose to create vibrant health for ourselves, we are enriching the quality of life on planet Earth as a whole, for at one level we are all connected—each person is a wave in this ocean of life. When you or I choose to be a responsible, loving, forgiving, healthy, happy person, living from integrity and oneness, this has a positive influence around the world, adding to the Light. By the same token, choosing the opposite decreases the world's light and wholeness. Each of us makes a difference by how we live. Marianne Williamson put it beautifully: "As we receive God's love and impart it to others, we are given the power to repair the world."

So if you take responsibility, acknowledge the sacredness of your body and life and walk a path with heart, greater world harmony will be created. Have faith in your vision, and your experience of living will become all the more magical and fulfilling. You will know what it means to be as you were created to be. Life will become an adventure, filled with celebration and joy. Wisdom, Love, and Light will be your constant companions. You will know serenity. You will become peace itself. It's your choice. Create vibrant health and bring serenity and sacred balance into your body and life, today and always.

The Joy factor

10 SACRED PRACTICES FOR RADIANT HEALTH

AUTHOR'S NOTE

The health suggestions and recommendations in this book are based on the training, research, and personal experiences of the author. Because each person and situation is unique, the author and publisher encourage the reader to check with his or her holistic physician or other health professional before using any procedure outlined in this book. It is a sign of wisdom to seek a second or third opinion. Neither the author nor the publisher is responsible for any adverse consequences resulting from a change in diet or from the use of any other suggestions in this book.

CHAPTER 1

Set the Bar High
I CHOOSE TO LIVE MY BEST LIFE

Whether you think you can or not, you are right.
–HENRY FORD

My business is not to remake myself,
but make the absolute best of what God made.
–ROBERT BROWNING

Just for a moment, close your eyes, breathe slowly and deeply a few times, and imagine yourself as the master of the universe. As master you have the ability to create anything you want, even something that has never existed before. Be adventurous in your thinking, focusing on the result and not just the means, and envision what you most want now.

You have this power within you—it is the birthright and potential of every human being. The only possible limitation is your own thought, belief, and imagination. Once you have a clear vision of what you want, then the natural play of universal forces will lead you to the accomplishment of that goal. Don't take your power lightly. Henry Ford knew all about it when he wrote, "Whether you think you can or not, you are right." You, and only you, have the ability to create miracles in your mind and life. The choice is always with you. It has nothing to do with luck and everything to do with believing in yourself as a part of the Divine Force that infuses and permeates everything in the universe. The great rule is this: if you can conceive it in your mind, then it can be brought into the physical world.

It takes boldness to go after your dreams, especially when you are exploring uncharted territory, but don't give up. In her perceptive book *Anatomy of the Spirit*, Caroline Myss warns that when you compromise your dreams and values to live a life that is expected of you, rather than what your heart asks of you, you give away your power and disconnect from your soul.

"It takes a lot of courage to release the familiar and seemingly secure, to embrace the new," says my friend Alan Cohen, author of *Handle with Prayer*. "But there is no real security in what is no longer meaningful. There is more security in the adventurous and exciting, for in movement there is life, and in change there is power."

The world today certainly offers change, and it's easy to regard ability to keep up with the changes, perhaps even to cause changes here and there, as power. But power is drained, not created, by surviving in such a fast-paced world. The intense pace and stress of our daily lives can very easily put our peace, happiness, and health—not to mention our spiritual lives—at risk. When we're caught up in the whirl of today's hectic lifestyle, it's easy to forget the truth of our potential. We have less and less time for our own dreams, and in such circumstances our standards and values tend to deteriorate, leading to low self-esteem. It is when we feel that kind of inner emptiness that we are most tempted by any "quick fix" that comes along.

Life is hard, and learning to live with sacredness takes time, but the fact is that we can slow things down. We can face our own challenges, however large or small, with aplomb and equanimity, on our own terms. We can choose to experience aliveness and become masters of our lives. My hope is that this book will point the way.

In the 1960s, psychologist Abraham Maslow wrote his famous *Toward a Psychology of Being*, which helped to change the entire emphasis of psychology. He chose to study high-functioning people —those living their highest potential—rather than people with problems, as was usually the case in psychology. Maslow developed a "psychology of being," which meant not striving but arriving, not trying to get someplace but living fully. Among all his high-functioning subjects, he found a common denominator. They all had a vision and were committed to it. They were self-motivated and believed they had the power to master life. That's one of the beliefs we will be working on throughout this book.

Do you believe you have the power to master life?

IF IT'S TO BE, IT'S UP TO ME

Self-mastery begins with a complete and honest inventory of our lives (see the workbook in Appendix A). As Socrates so famously said, "The unexamined life is not worth living." Mastery involves taking responsibility for ourselves and what we've created, rather than blaming other people and circumstances for our lot in life. Blame is a convenient way of explaining why our life is not exactly what we would like it to be. The next time you start to blame another person or outside circumstances for how you feel or what you are experiencing, stop, check yourself, and remember: What you feel is up to you. Our feelings are governed by our mind. We can't think one thing and feel something else. Feelings and experiences always correspond to thoughts. If you are to become master of your life and live your highest potential, the habit of blaming others or circumstances has to stop. Setbacks and obstacles are only tests.

Mastery involves being self-disciplined and courageous, moving through fear, recognizing our inherent Divine Power, and using it to bring our vision to life. Millions of masters-in-the-making, like you and me, are awakening to the concepts of self-responsibility and choice. The proof is in the success of teachers such as Louise L. Hay, Oprah, Ellen DeGeneres, Wayne Dyer, Mehmet Oz, Deepak Chopra, Suze Orman, and others who help people bring spirituality and wholeness into everyday life. Once introduced to these empowering ideas, people give up being victims in favor of being masters. Self-mastery means becoming the heroes of our own lives.

Instead of whining "Why?" and pointing the finger of blame, masters say, "This is the situation. I take responsibility for it. I realize I created this emotional stuff. I know I have the power to make new choices about how I view any event and how I react to it. I am powerful enough to 'uncreate' this situation and re-create something healthy and joyful. I now choose to see everything through the eyes of Love."

Love empowers us. Nothing will transform and enrich life faster than the consistent experience of Love. Let others know that you love them. Tell them and show them, often. Don't wait until later, for you don't know if they will still be here tomorrow. Paramahansa Yogananda used to say that if we want to live our highest potential, all we have to do is teach the mind how to think differently—how to be gentle, calm, loving, and centered on God. Seeing through the eyes of Love is the same as seeing through the eyes of God. Become comfortable with the idea that you are a spiritual being in a physical body, live from that awareness moment to moment, and your life will be transformed. It's simply an internal shift—a journey of mere inches from your mind to your heart. You will find yourself more certain, fulfilled, successful, content, and peaceful than ever before. You will be living in a state of grace.

Anyone who goes about living with a sense of serenity, contentment, and grace has no need to manipulate others. It is rare for a person who is reasonably satisfied with his or her own life to try to run someone else's. Such a person continues to grow through a living process of discovery and renewal and finds that self-mastery is the very opposite of control. As paradoxical as it may sound, this is the path to self-mastery: to surrender, trust, turn away from habits of accumulation, outer achievement, and quick fixes, and to allow one's sense of purpose to spring from inner guidance.

The more you live from inner guidance—that peaceful, loving center within you—the more you'll find that everything you need to meet your wants and desires will be provided. The essence is in knowing that you are already whole and that nothing external to yourself in the physical world can make you any more complete.

YOUR REALITY REFLECTS YOUR THOUGHTS AND INTENTIONS

We create our thoughts, our thoughts create our intentions, and our intentions create our reality. What you see around you, whom you associate with, how you function daily, what your relationships are like, how much money you make, how you get along with others, the shape of your physical body, and virtually everything about you is the result of your intention. Intention is directional energy, and intentional living is one of the most empowering ways to achieve happiness, health, and wholeness and to banish obstacles to spiritual growth. When life is lived with conscious intention, insights unfold more easily and everything proceeds more gracefully.

It is usually fairly easy to be happy and peaceful and to feel somewhat saintly when removed from social circumstances and relationships, but to be happy, peaceful, and balanced regardless of personal and environmental conditions is evidence of real spiritual growth. As you become more soul-centered, your personal and environmental reality tends to adjust toward harmony. Your intentions reflect your values and higher spiritual Self back out into the world. If you view the world as a giving place, you probably see goodness in others and in all situations and are optimistic about other people's being kind and considerate. You usually find yourself surrounded by others with similar values. As a natural result, you experience much gratitude and are unconsciously teaching others to be more loving.

Our main job here on Earth is to take our focus and attention off criticizing and finding fault, and instead look for ways to serve others, share the peace and joy of our hearts, and let others know we appreciate them. When we continually find fault with someone, he or she withers up like a flower without water. Show love, respect, and appreciation to others and they will blossom. Isn't that what we all want—simply to be loved and appreciated?

Give this a try: for a day or two, treat others as if the fullness of God resided within them. Imagine that their external attributes are nonexistent and that you can look directly into their hearts.

In any relationship with others, what really matters is the heart-to-heart or love connection. At the level of the heart, we are all connected by love, yet the love that connects us also makes us complete and whole beings within ourselves. The secret of relationships, whether they are with lovers, friends, or business associates, is to maintain our individuality in union. Remember that you are two selves. Let the winds of heaven dance between you always. Let Spirit guide you. The essence of who you are is Spirit. Spirit makes us all equally special and precious.

Being master of my life means that I put God first before everything. I choose to do this, trusting that my life's higher purpose is being revealed to me. My connection to God requires that I live my highest and best at all times and in all circumstances. I know the loving presence will give me the strength and courage to follow through on my commitments. Being centered on God also means that I give up depending on people, circumstances, and material things as my sources of happiness and fulfillment. I choose to put my faith in God and in my inner guidance.

SUCCESS IS AN INSIDE JOB

For years I have done research on what makes people successful. I recently learned about Daniel Isenberg, a professor at the Harvard Business School and a very popular teacher. He said that for years his former students would come back to him and say, "We really liked your courses, but now that we're out in the real world, what we learned at the business school doesn't seem to make much sense."

This bothered Isenberg because he wanted to teach his students something useful. So he obtained the names of the 25 most successful executives in the country and got permission to follow each of them around for a week, to find out what it was they did that made them successful. Isenberg listened to their phone conversations, listened to them talk to their colleagues, friends, and families, and came to the conclusion that what made these people successful had nothing to do with what was taught at the business school. He discovered two important characteristics shared by all the successful people he observed.

One thing these achievers had in common was a commitment to putting their values first. There may come a time in our lives when our goals are in conflict with our values, a time when we want to do something in business or in some other connection, but we know it's a little judgmental or even a little unethical. We find ourselves torn between what we want to do at the moment and what we feel or know is right. What Isenberg's group of successful people had in common was loyalty to their values. They had learned that, without commitment to our values, either we don't achieve our goals, or if we do, they're not really worth achieving after all.

The second thing these highly successful executives had in common was an incredible faith in their intuition. They all exhibited spiritual sensibility. Some of them were churchgoers, some were not, but they all had a sense of a deeper intelligence in the universe that operated through them. Each of these people made decisions based on his intuitive feelings about what was going on in his business or professional life. We are all endowed with this "sixth sense" of intuition, but most people seem to rely on the other five senses, which usually interpret things according to their own likes and dislikes rather than according to what is true and beneficial for the soul. To know how to choose correctly in any given situation, we need to let the power of intuition guide our judgments.

How in tune are you with your intuition—with God's whisperings?

THE ROLE OF THE BODY IN SELF-MASTERY

Living our best life means appreciating our magnificent bodies. The body is sacred, a temple of the living, loving spirit, and therefore deserves reverence. Treat yourself with respect. Don't wait until you're sick to recognize the miracle of your body. Honor the love inside you and the love you are. If you want to become healthier and more powerful, begin with how you feel about yourself, accepting your body as a temple. Heaven on Earth is inside each one of us at this moment. In your unique body, mind, and spirit you have been given everything you need to be the best you can be, to become master of your life. Cherish and respect your body unconditionally—no matter what its current shape—because it is sacred.

As Divine beings, we all deserve tender, loving care. We may find this difficult to accept, especially where our bodies are concerned. Many of us need to learn to be a friend to our bodies. Getting angry with our bodies only makes matters worse. Although they are but temporary homes for our spiritual being, we must still take care of them because they are sacred vessels for this voyage on Earth. Love your body and be committed to staying fit for your life journey.

Start today by tuning in more attentively to your body. It is a fantastic feedback machine. If you listen, you will discover that it communicates very well. When you get a headache, your body is trying to tell you something. Listen to your body's signals. The key is your willingness to listen and act. If you feel pain, what is your body trying to tell you? It may be telling you that you're eating too much, or eating the wrong kinds of food, or smoking or drinking too much, or not sleeping enough, or not drinking enough water or getting enough exercise. It could be telling you that there's too much emotional congestion in your life.

Listen to your body. Respect and appreciate it. Take loving care of it. You will learn to discern what your body is trying to tell you. And please, choose your doctor carefully. Choose someone who practices a wellness lifestyle and who listens to you. There is a tendency today for doctors to turn to technology and all kinds of elaborate testing, or to prescribe a regimen of medications, before listening to you or to their own intuition. I don't think it's a positive trend. As you think about your health and health care, ask yourself both of these questions: "What can the doctor do for me?" and "How can I help myself?" You are the authority on your body. Educate yourself. If you have specific health conditions, read up on them online and figure out how to get the best possible care. And remember this: It is normal to be healthy. It's your divine birthright to be well.

LOVE IS THE MAIN INGREDIENT TO BEING MASTER OF YOUR HEALTH

One of the most powerful things you can do for your health is to love yourself unconditionally, every day. Treat yourself with respect and dignity. These are the simplest ways to experience peace and the joy of living. It may sound too simple, but I urge you to consider the power of self-love. Remind yourself constantly, so you won't forget. Stick notes on the refrigerator and the mirrors around your home if you need to. "I love myself." "I treat myself with the utmost dignity." Erich Fromm said, "Our highest calling in life is precisely to take loving care of ourselves." When you change your attitude about yourself from negative to positive, everything else in your life will change for the better.

One of the extraordinary secrets of this world is that life flows outward. It originates inside and is projected outward, where it is perceived as the external world. People and situations and circumstances don't affect us unless we allow them to. We are affected only by what happens inside us, how we process situations, interactions, and events. We are affected only by our own feelings and our own thoughts. Nothing outside has the power to affect us.

When you change your attitude about yourself from negative to

positive, everything else in your life will change for the better.

Most people denigrate themselves all the time, in fun or in earnest. Beware, because in doing that, especially out loud or publicly, you create your own problems. If you think that somebody else hurts you or makes you happy or that some other person makes you feel good or bad about yourself, it's a delusion. Nobody else is responsible for your pain or pleasure. Nobody else is responsible for your sorrow or joy. You are the only one who can change what you think and how you feel. Make it a personal policy never to put yourself down. Never debase yourself or think negatively about yourself. Tune in to the inner guidance that is with you 24/7 and realize that you are whole and wonderful and powerful beyond measure.

When you get in touch with your innermost Self and come in contact with that infinite, invisible intelligence that is always a part of you and your daily life, you know what you should think, do, and say. Embrace your feelings—all of them. Pay attention to what your body, mind, and heart are telling you. You are getting messages all the time. For example, let's say you have made a commitment to only speak and think positive words and thoughts about yourself and your body. Then you find yourself walking by a store window and you see a reflection of your body in the window. The distortion of the glass expands your size. For a moment you cringe, and then your internal voice starts blathering out denigrations such as "I'll never be able to get down to my ideal weight" or "If only I had smaller hips and thighs" or "I wish I looked like the women on the TV show *Desperate Housewives*" or "That's it, I'm so depressed at how I look today that I think I'll wait until next Monday to start fresh and will just eat whatever I want for the rest of this week." When something like this happens, focus directly on what is right in front of you, your goal, and the truth of your being. Bring your thoughts back to the positive. Direct your attention to the things you appreciate about yourself and your body. When any experience keeps repeating, this is a signal demanding further attention.

Don't be afraid of darkness, of dark or negative feelings, for darkness is the harbinger of light. "The dark night of the soul," says Joseph Campbell, "comes just before revelation. When everything is lost and all seems darkest, then comes the new life and all that is needed." In other words, sometimes things need to fall apart in our lives in order to come together again and unfold at a higher level. To make that happen, turn everything in your life over to the divinity within you. That Divine Self, that Light and Love within you, exists within everybody but is being wasted by those who don't take the time to turn within. You may not find it easy at first, but everybody can do it with practice.

For example, even though you might have recently made a commitment to create more prosperity in your life, or meet new friends, or detox your body, it's not uncommon for the "appearances" in those specific areas to seem to get worse. In fact, when you're detoxifying, your body goes through a house-cleansing and you might experience a few days of feeling worse before you feel better. If you choose to say hello to strangers on the street or at office or social gatherings, you might experience many cold shoulders before you find a tenderhearted person with whom you would like to create a friendship. I always look at everything as Spirit's way to keep me heading in the right direction. I trust that everything will unfold perfectly when I keep my intentions and goals directly in front of me.

DIVINITY IS ANOTHER MAIN INGREDIENT

A most useful way to begin each day is with prayer and meditation.

I urge you to make meditation a top priority in your life. Don't mystify it. The process of meditation is nothing more than quietly going within and discovering your highest self. Meditation also allows you to empty yourself of the endless activity of your mind and to attain calmness. Regular meditation has many benefits. It is a natural way to attain peace of mind: it strengthens the body's immune system, slows the biologic aging process, awakens regenerative energies, enlivens the nervous system, and enhances creative abilities. Meditation will enable you to be more peaceful, soul-centered, and aware of the spiritual dimensions of your life. With progressive spiritual growth, you will be more insightful and more intellectually and intuitively capable of discerning the difference between truth and untruth. Ultimately, when you adopt meditation as a way of life, you'll be able to go to that peaceful place within yourself anytime and carry that peace and joy to all the circumstances in your life.

Meditation is a natural way to attain peace of mind. It strengthens the body's immune system, slows the biologic aging process, awakens regenerative energies, enlivens the nervous system, and enhances creative abilities.

Listen to Franz Kafka: "You do not need to leave your room. Remain sitting at your table and listen. Do not even listen, simply wait. Do not even wait, be quiet, still and solitary. The world will freely offer itself to you to be unmasked, it has no choice; it will roll in ecstasy at your feet."

Once you make a routine of daily spiritual practice, look for the proof of its value in how you live every waking moment. It is in the arena of everyday circumstances and relationships that we are provided with opportunities to explore the depth and clarity of our understanding.

How we experience life is a direct reflection of our inner condition, of our psychological health, maturity, understanding of our reason for living, and willingness to do what it takes to live successfully.

As important as it is to develop a spiritual practice, it is equally important not to become addicted to it or to indulge yourself in inner work to the exclusion of meaningful activities and relationships. Be sure to balance your regular sessions of meditation, inner reflection, and prayer with worthwhile involvements in your outer life. In this way you fulfill yourself and your purpose in life.

If this all sounds high minded, remember this: It doesn't matter if you've never done it before. It doesn't matter what your level of health or spirituality is right now. At any moment you can choose differently. You can use your past mistakes or poor choices and learn from them. In fact, some people have to be at the very bottom before they awaken to the fact that they can choose something else. This is exactly what happened to a friend of mine, Mary June.

MARY JUNE'S TRANSFORMATION

As the sun was shining over Santa Monica Bay, with its panoply of luscious colors illuminating the sky and the water, I was skating on the bike path, oblivious to people playing on the beach or passing by me. Alone and pensive, caught up in the fluid motion of my body and mind harmoniously in sync, I felt a palpable peacefulness—so often fleeting in today's stress-filled lives—infusing every cell in my body and permeating my thoughts. The melodious syncopation of the waves caressing the sand accompanied each stride.

And then it happened. What felt like a gigantic rock—it was actually only a quarter-sized stone—caught a wheel of my in-line skate and down I went, slamming into the cement. Fortunately, at that moment no one was there to see my less-than-graceful descent, except for a woman sitting on a bench about ten feet away. She immediately came over to make sure I was okay. Her gentle kindness and amiable countenance immediately comforted me. She helped me to the bench, where I removed my helmet. When I saw the jagged lacerations on the helmet, I felt overjoyed and grateful that I had worn protection and that nothing in my body was broken—just a few minor scratches and abrasions on my arms and legs and some major bruises to my ego.

As I got myself under control and determined that I could skate back to my car, I focused my attention on the sympathetic woman by my side and noticed from her swollen, bloodshot eyes that she had been crying. Feeling I could help, I invited her, after exchanging a few niceties, to have lunch with me, and she acquiesced. So I skated to my car and we met a few minutes later at a nearby restaurant.

We all have difficult and sometimes heartbreaking stories to tell, and Mary June (MJ) was no exception. Over a three-hour lunch I learned, in a nutshell, that MJ's two children had been killed by a drunk driver less than a year before. Soon thereafter she discovered that her husband was having an affair with his assistant, who was 25 years his junior. He had recently served her with divorce papers—just weeks after they had learned she had breast cancer. Then, a couple of days before we met, she had been let go from her job because of all the time she had been absent from work, owing to the necessity for medical care.

Through all the twists and turns of her recent life, MJ had kept a remarkably optimistic attitude and ability to rise above her challenges and had been able to hold onto a childlike trust and belief that there had to be some Divine order to it all. I learned that only minutes before my fall, sadness had overcome her and she had been crying, grieving the loss of her family and husband, her breast, her job, and everything about the normal life she thought was hers only a year before. It would have been easy to see herself as a victim and sink into despair, and most people she knew would not have blamed her, but MJ believed there was another, better way.

Fortunately, MJ had enough money to live for a few months without needing to work. Her only goal now was to create a healthy, balanced lifestyle and find ways to nurture her body, mind, and spirit. She told me that she wanted to lose weight and get back into shape, simplify the clutter in her house and beautify her surroundings, learn to meditate, plant a garden, and find some good books to read to nurture her new holistic lifestyle, but she didn't know where to start.

At that moment I discovered why my angels had made me fall practically at her feet. Until then, she was not aware of my work, books, and passion for motivating others to live their highest vision. When she found out about what I did and that I was giving a three-hour workshop that same evening called "Celebrate Life: Rejuvenate Body, Mind & Spirit with Empowering Disciplines," we both laughed until we cried. What a providential encounter it was, and what a powerful lesson for both of us that we're always in the right place at the right time and are constantly being guided and cared for by a loving Presence. Only minutes before I crashed into her world, she was asking God for the right direction to take and the best person to guide her in living a more healthy, balanced lifestyle.

Over the next three months, I was MJ's holistic lifestyle coach. We started by writing out her goals and dreams and creating affirmations to support her highest vision for herself. She immediately implemented a well-rounded exercise regime, which included aerobics, strength training, and flexibility exercises. In her home, we started with the kitchen and cleaned out anything and everything that wasn't for her highest good, nearly emptying the cupboards, pantry, and refrigerator. We went shopping at the local health food store and the supermarket so that she'd have healthy foods in her home from which to choose.

Next, we cleaned out every drawer and closet in her home (my passion for simplifying, organizing, and beautifying our surroundings has resulted in a fulfilling side business I call "Simply Organized"), added cheerful shelf paper here and there, and brightened some walls with new paint. We extended the theme of brightening and adding more color by creating two lovely gardens in the front and back of her home, where nothing but weeds had grown. As an amateur horticulturist and landscape designer, I relish getting my hands in the soil, planting a variety of greenery, flowers, and trees, and working with the nature angels to create a natural, celestial environment that will attract birds—especially hummingbirds—and butterflies. I even persuaded MJ to add a fountain to her yard and bring a couple more into her home as a way of fostering tranquility and serenity. Finally, I taught her how to meditate, a discipline she took to like a butterfly to buddleia (a butterfly-loving plant!).

MJ made a conscious choice to surrender her life to God and commit herself to being the best she could be. Within six months, she was down to her ideal weight, having lost 33 pounds, and was fitter and healthier than she had ever been in her life. After taking a few classes in interior design, a dream of hers since she was young, she started working part-time as an assistant to a prominent designer in Santa Monica. Because of her courage and assiduity, her healthy diet, a positive and balanced lifestyle that nurtures her body, mind, and spirit, and a support team of doctors and friends, MJ feels confident that neither cancer nor any other degenerative disease will ever be part of her life again. And when she least expected it—as she was working out in the gym—she met a loving, upstanding man who shares many of her interests and has asked her to go with him on a long trip to Europe.

I have no doubt that our meeting was divinely guided for our mutual empowerment. I helped her transform and enhance her life; MJ profoundly inspired and motivated me with her integrity, willing spirit, and devotion to making her life better. She realized that "If it's to be, it's up to me" and took responsibility for her own happiness and fulfillment. She has discovered her purpose, followed her heart, and begun living with authentic power and passion. MJ and I both learned firsthand that breakthroughs and miracles occur when we're willing to live our vision and commitment.

THE POWER OF COMMITMENT

Lack of commitment is like an epidemic in our society. Just look around. People say they're committed to creating a healthier, more harmonious planet, yet they continue to litter, don't recycle, and drive cars that pollute. They say they're committed to their relationships, yet they lie, are unfaithful, are unwilling to be vulnerable, or walk out at the first sign of difficulty or challenge. They say they're committed to aligning with the spiritual side of their natures, but they set aside no time for meditation, solitude, or communion with our higher power.

Many people wish they felt more committed and wish they had something really big to commit to. They don't realize that the first big commitment has to be to themselves. By really committing to your best self and following through on your convictions and decisions, you will gain tremendous power. Nothing can keep you from becoming master of your life.

When you're committed to your health, you allow nothing to deter you from reaching your goal and are disciplined even when you're not feeling motivated. Discipline is the ability to carry out a resolution long after the mood and enthusiasm have left you. Of course there were times when MJ didn't feel like making a healthy dinner or getting up early to exercise after she had stayed up late to see a movie or visit friends, but she harnessed that inner commitment and persisted in keeping her word to herself. And on those few occasions when she experienced setbacks, instead of beating herself up with guilt and anger for doing something unhealthy, she came to see that these were choices from which she could learn and perhaps make better ones the next time. As she began to pay close attention, she noticed that binging on unhealthy food made her feel lethargic for the next few days, and she quickly came to realize that the momentary taste pleasure wasn't worth hours and days of feeling sluggish and morose. This is how we change: by paying attention and by our commitments.

Discipline is the ability to carry out a resolution long after the mood and enthusiasm have left you.

When we make a commitment, we are willing to put all of our resources on the line and take responsibility for the outcome. Commitment—to a project, a relationship, or a health and fitness program—brings stability to the chaotic whirl of everyday life. Daily acts that reaffirm the commitment will increase our feelings of empowerment and self-esteem. The better MJ felt about herself, the more easily she made choices that were for her highest good, like going to the gym earlier than usual some mornings because of a busy schedule, or like choosing to eat more colorful, plant-based foods and drink more water and fresh juice even when she yearned to eat something unhealthy.

Through our everyday behavior we learn what really counts. Commitment, like peacefulness, must be woven through all of life, through our thoughts, emotions, words, and actions. I often hear people say they are committed to being healthy, yet they continually let things get in the way. They say they'll have to wait "until next Monday or the day after" to exercise because they're "just too busy now," even though they've made a commitment to exercise every day. Or they won't be able to start eating nutritious meals for the next two weeks because of birthdays, anniversaries, travels, or because they are "just too stressed out" to make a major change right now.

Commitment means that you get past your excuses and follow through on what you said you were going to do. Make your word count, especially your word to yourself. How can you ever expect someone else to make a commitment to you, and how can they ever expect you to follow through on a commitment to them, unless you show that you can keep a commitment to yourself? If you are committed, you arrange your personal circumstances so that your lifestyle supports your commitment. You can and will do whatever it takes to put your life in order, let go of excess baggage and nonessentials, and consciously focus on what is important.

TURN ADVERSITY TO ADVANTAGE

In my life and the lives of many people I know, the most growth, the greatest lessons, and the most rewarding transformations have always sprung from the greatest adversities and challenges. MJ's experience is a perfect example. If we haven't worked through or learned from these challenges, they have a way of reappearing in more damaging form. But once we've heeded the message and committed to changing our course, life has a way of making certain past misfortunes pay extra dividends. I'll bet you know exactly what I mean.

Here's an example from my life: A few years ago I signed a multi-book contract with a major book publisher. The second book in the series needed to be written more quickly than was comfortable for my balanced living lifestyle. It meant that I needed to curtail all socializing for over three months while I focused on writing the book and on my other work responsibilities. I explained the situation to my friends and told them that I would only be able to see them if they were willing to come with me on my early morning hikes. Well, very few (in fact only two) friends agreed to visit with me early mornings, but they did end up accompanying me regularly for sunrise hikes. These visits turned out to be the highlight of my week. We discussed issues I was addressing in the book, which in turn made it much easier to write when I sat down at my computer. During this same period I was invited to appear on a prestigious national television talk show. It would have required a few days of travel and work, and I didn't see how I could take that kind of time away from my writing. When I thanked the producer and asked her to check back with me in two months, she just laughed. She thought I was joking.

For days, I was filled with doubt, wondering if I had made a big mistake. But life, as I say, has a way of rewarding us for taking care of ourselves. Once the book was released, I sent it to the same producer. She called immediately and offered me an even greater TV opportunity. She also told me that she applauded my commitment to my goal and how I let nothing stand in the way of bringing it to fruition. She said that my decision to forego her first TV offer gave her pause and ended up being a catalyst for her to be more focused in her work and personal commitments. In fact, those were some of the very topics that we discussed on the TV show when I finally arrived and participated.

Blaming, complaining, and taking no action only keeps us in a rut. It is important to always look beyond how a situation appears and to choose to see our lives from a higher perspective. The secret is to view everything around you as an aspect of yourself. In this way you shatter the illusion of separation and with it the need to blame and complain.

If you are feeling stuck, ask this question: What is it I need to learn to finish this business so I can move on in my life? Choose to turn adversity into opportunity by taking responsibility for everything you've created in your life and accepting the consequences of your choices, both good and bad. It gets you nowhere to transfer blame to other people or circumstances. You must be willing to accept whatever happens as the product of your own thoughts and actions.

Accepting responsibility can feel very burdensome and scary, I know. When I began taking responsibility for everything I was or wasn't creating in my life, I was scared. If my life wasn't working, I had no one to blame but myself, and that felt awful at first. But soon I realized that taking responsibility was also very empowering and freeing. I could steer this ship any way I wanted!

This is what living is all about—mastering our lives by becoming all that we were created to be.

Try to avoid making routine matters and everyday relationships complicated. Your life is your gift to yourself and to the world through thoughtful service to others. Knowing this, I encourage you to unfailingly and enthusiastically welcome each day with joy and thankfulness because of the limitless opportunity it offers to learn, grow, flourish, and be truly happy and fulfilled, even—no, especially—if it feels hard to do. If this approach to each new day is not already a habit with you, make it your first priority from now on. Practice the presence of Spirit.

Look deep within yourself to get in touch with the truth of your being and the unlimited possibilities that await you. To assist in the process, you may want to ponder these questions and thoughts, as I had MJ do at the start of her commitment program.

PERSONAL COMMITMENT STATEMENT

Complete—on paper—the following statements. They will give you some insight about how to use the Self-Discovery Questions and Action Choices in Appendix A:

- This is how my life would be if I were now living my highest vision:
- I commit to do the following to make my vision my reality:
- These are the ways I will now rearrange my lifestyle in order to support my commitments:
- The non-useful behaviors I will discontinue are:
- The new, constructive behaviors I will implement are:
- I will nurture my spiritual self by:

Write out the following Personal Commitment Statement at the bottom of your answers and read it out loud and with feeling. Sign your name, and date it. Reread it often. This is a positive personal commitment for everybody. From time to time, as you achieve your goals and live your vision at higher levels, you will want to rewrite and refine your Personal Commitment Statement.

I am passionately, unshakably devoted to my vision of how I want my life to be. I am committed to making my vision a reality, for I know I have the power and ability to live my vision. Everything unlike my vision is dissipating, easily and effortlessly. I agree and affirm that I will do my best to help myself to total wellness and spiritual growth, and I will share my increasing radiance with my world. What I sincerely desire for myself I also see and allow for others. Thank you for this precious gift of life. Today, as always, I honor and serve Spirit by loving myself and everyone else unconditionally and by acknowledging Spirit's presence in everything I think, feel, say, and do.

MAKE A DIFFERENCE

You can make a profound difference in other people's lives by the way you choose to live yours. I'm reminded of the story of a young boy who was walking down the beach, picking up starfish, and throwing them out into the waves. A man watched him for a while and finally caught up with the youth. He asked, "What are you doing that for?" The boy answered that the stranded starfish would die if left in the morning sun. "But the beach goes on for miles and there are millions of starfish," countered the man. "How can your effort make any difference?" The boy looked at the starfish in his hand, threw it hard back into the sea, and replied, "It made a difference to that one!"

It makes a difference to those around you when you are loving, peaceful, happy, and healthy. It makes a difference every place you go when you are master of your life. You make a difference.

Our bodies are made up of billions of cells. In order to maintain optimum health, each of these cells must operate at peak performance. When we have sick or weak cells, the stronger, healthier ones must work harder so that our body as a whole will be healthy. Consider that the human race is like a body, and we are each its individual cells. If we are all cells in the same body, then ultimately we are not separate from others. There is no room for negative thinking, lack of forgiveness, hubris, bitterness towards others, or selfishness. It is our responsibility to this global body to be a healthy, happy, peaceful, loving cell that radiates only goodness, positivity, and joy. Think of it as contributing to the health and harmony of the whole world.

For too long, our thoughts and beliefs regarding our life on this planet have been colored by artificial divisions. It is time we examined and corrected them. To create peace on Earth, we must stop dividing the world—the nations, the races, the religions, the sexes, the ages, the families, and the resources—and realize it is time to live together in peace, forgiveness, and love. Awareness that we are one must precede all our thoughts and actions as a part of our belief system. We are all connected to one another and to this living, breathing planet. We have a choice, and we can choose to make a difference with the way we live our lives.

In his book *The Hundredth Monkey*, Ken Keyes, Jr., tells of a phenomenon observed by scientists. The eating habits of macaque monkeys were studied on several islands. One monkey discovered that sweet potatoes tasted better when she washed them before eating them. That monkey taught her mother and friends until one day a certain number (ninety-nine, to be exact) of the monkeys knew how to wash their sweet potatoes. The next day, when the hundredth monkey learned how to wash sweet potatoes, an amazing thing happened: the rest of the colony miraculously knew how to wash their sweet potatoes, too! Not only that, but the monkeys on other islands started washing their sweet potatoes as well. Strange, but true.

Keyes applies this "hundredth monkey" phenomenon to humanity. When more of us individually choose to make a difference with our lives—when human beings realize we each make a difference and start acting as though we do—more and more of us will learn this truth until we reach the "millionth person," and peace and cooperation will spread across the globe. I believe that, although we can't change the world, we can choose to know and change ourselves and that as we do, the world will be different. We will truly be masters of the universe—not by controlling one another, but by being masters of ourselves all together.

We're here on Earth not to see through one another, but to see one another through. We are here to experience the fullness of life. We are here to become the best we can be. We owe it to ourselves. As we change ourselves, we change the world. At a sermon that I attended, the late Unity minister and author Eric Butterworth said, "It is not so much ours to set the world right, rather it is ours to see it rightly."

If you can think of yourself as being all that you know you should be: constant, gentle, loving and kind to every man, woman, and child, and to every circumstance in life; kind and tolerant in your attitude towards all conditions on earth;

Above all, if you can conceive yourself as being completely calm in all conditions and circumstances, quiet and yet strong—strong to aid your weaker brethren, strong to speak the right word, to take the right action, and so become a tower of strength and light;

If you can see yourself facing injustice and unkindness with a serene spirit, knowing that all things work out in time for good, and that justice is always eventually triumphant;

If you have patience to await the process of the outworking of the will of God; if you can picture becoming like this, you will know something of mastership.
—White Eagle, The Quiet Mind

There is only one journey. Going inside yourself.
—Rainer Maria Rilke

Just trust yourself; then you will know how to live.
—Johann Wolfgang von Goethe

CHAPTER 2

Act with Kindness

I CHOOSE TO SPREAD HAPPINESS WHEREVER I GO

Of course I love everyone I meet. How could I fail to do so?
Within everyone is the spark of God. I am not concerned
with racial or ethnic background or the color of one's skin;
all people look to me like shining lights!
—PEACE PILGRIM

To find your own way is to follow your own bliss. This involves analysis,
watching yourself, and seeing where the real deep bliss is—not the quick
little excitement, but the real, deep, life-filling bliss.
—JOSEPH CAMPBELL

I could hear the frustration in her voice the moment I picked up the telephone. My friend Rose called me because she was on the verge of quitting her job, even though she loved her work. She needed some guidance.

Rose is a very talented window dresser for a popular store on Rodeo Drive in Beverly Hills. She loves what she does, but she had been having an extremely difficult time with her boss. During our conversation, she told me how often she felt that some of her best work was rejected and unappreciated by her supervisor. Not only were most of his criticisms unjustified, she said, but she was convinced he was deliberately rude and unfair to her. Because I believe we always attract to ourselves the equivalent of what we think, feel, and believe, I lovingly suggested to my friend that maybe she, rather than her boss, was the one in need of an attitude adjustment. Besides, she couldn't change him; the only person she could change was herself. The attitudes we harbor can harden to block our perspective on everything and foil discovering our bliss. I asked her how she felt about him.

Rose confessed that her mind was filled with criticism and unkindness toward this man and that she rarely felt positive in his presence because of the way he treated her. She even revealed to me that every morning as she walked to work, she would visualize the entire scenario of how badly he would act toward her that day. Rose confirmed my observation about the law of correspondence. I explained to her that he was merely bearing witness to her conception of him.

When Rose realized what she had been doing, she agreed to change her attitude and think of her boss only in a kind, loving way. I recommended that, before drifting off to sleep at night, she visualize him congratulating her on her fine designs and creativity and that she see herself, in turn, thanking him for his support and kindness. To her delight, after she had practiced her visualizations for only seven days, the behavior of her employer miraculously reversed itself. Rose proved the power of imagination and kindness. Her commitment to replace unkindness with love and openheartedness influenced his behavior as much as it did hers and reshaped his attitude toward her. If he hadn't changed his behavior, I know that Rose would have eventually found another job that utilized her creative gifts and talents in an environment where she was validated, appreciated, and cherished. We don't know we have this power until we try it, but it is always the same—as within, so without.

Humans are powerful spiritual beings who can create good on the Earth. This good isn't usually accomplished in bold actions but in modest acts of kindness and love between people. The little things do count, because they are more spontaneous and show who we truly are. Whatever amount of love and good feelings we feel at the end of our life is equal to the love and good feelings we put out during our life. It's that simple. "What a splendid way to move through the world," writes Jack Kornfield in *A Path with Heart*, "to bring our blessings to all that we touch. To honor, to bless, to welcome with the heart is never done in grand or monumental ways, but in this moment, in the most immediate and intimate way."

THE RELIGION OF KINDNESS

Antoine de Saint-Exupéry wrote in *The Little Prince* that "what's truly essential is invisible to the eye—it can only be seen and felt with the heart."

"When strangers start acting like neighbors, communities are reinvigorated," said Ralph Nader. Acts of kindness send out a positive ripple into the world and help bring us back to the feeling that people are basically good and kind. The love you give never runs out, for the more you share with others, the more you have to give.

The Dalai Lama would wholeheartedly agree. He says, "My religion is very simple—my religion is kindness." Kindness is an integral part of the choice to live fully. Not just kindness but gentleness. In my mind, they go hand-in-hand. Gentle means kindly, mild, and amiable—not violent or severe. Gentleness also implies compassion, consideration, tolerance, calmness, mild temper, courtesy, and peacefulness. But the word I like to think of in connection with gentle is tenderhearted. I feel instantly at home with people who are tenderhearted. What about you? Think about the people you love to be around the most, with whom you feel the most enthusiastic and positive and able to be yourself. You'll probably refer to them as loving, supportive, kind, and maybe even tenderhearted.

To be treated with tenderheartedness and kindness, you must first offer those qualities to other people. Think that others deserve exactly the same treatment you would like for yourself.

No one likes to be belittled, ignored, vituperated, or unappreciated. Everyone warms to kindness, patience, and respect.

I'll never forget the morning of January 17, 1994. It was 4:31 a.m. and I was in my home in Brentwood, Los Angeles, meditating on the floor in front of my altar. All of a sudden everything was in an uproar, and my first reaction was that God was speaking to me! Then I knew it was the biggest earthquake I had ever felt. I will never forget the terrifying sensation of hanging on to the corner of my bed while everything in my home crashed to the floor. It felt and sounded like the end of the world, and I was certain I was going to die. For almost everyone who went through the experience, it seemed as if the epicenter was right under their own home, and as if the duration was four minutes rather than 40 seconds. For those seconds and the hours that followed, I was living totally in the present moment.

But what's germane and important here is the response from the community. Adversity always brings gifts and powerful lessons. Our indomitable, munificent spirit rears up and unites us with one another. After the earthquake, families, friends, and even strangers reached out to one another with true tenderheartedness and kindness. Sharing the same experience brought people together on common (if shaky) ground and opened our hearts to one another. Southern California was invigorated with a new spirit of compassion.

Now that September 11, 2001 has brought the entire United States and much of the world together in feelings of loss, compassion, and generosity, our sense of oneness with those who suffer from any natural or man-made catastrophe may become stronger. So many have discovered that acts of kindness in and of themselves have amazing power to heal both those who receive them and those who perform them. Certainly this was true following the 1994 earthquake, when the crime rate in our area went to its lowest level in years. We were forced to slow down and to see more clearly what is really important in life: not the things we possess or even the work we do, but the people in our lives, the heart-to-heart connection we have with others, and the love we give.

Acts of kindness connect our heart to the heart of another person and create bridges over which our love can flow. Sometimes they are anonymous and sometimes not. Either way, they change us. When we give of our highest Selves purely out of love, our body, our heart, and our environment change, and for an instant we realize that loving and being loved is the one true human vocation. We feel connected to the love in ourselves and the love in others.

Don't ever underestimate the power of kindness. "Random acts of kindness" may just be a slogan, but it has caught on all around the country for a reason. Doing lovely things for others for no reason has so many rewards. In an instant, the best of our humanity and heart comes forward. Such gestures aren't expected, but every time we seize the opportunity to perform them, we are transformed. We become, in a sense, an angel for a moment and touch the Divine. By giving someone else pure love and joy without expecting something in return, we become twice blessed—in blessing another we also bless ourselves.

Every day presents us with hundreds of opportunities to practice kindness toward our fellow humans. Seize these moments and discover how wonderful it feels. Not long ago I was moved by a gesture of love at the airport. I was leaving Portland, Oregon, to fly to Los Angeles. Because of stormy weather, most flights were delayed, and some were canceled. The airport was crowded with unhappy travelers, so I was delighted that for some reason my flight was scheduled to leave on time. As they announced the final boarding, I noticed a harried man running up to the counter with his briefcase in one hand and his ticket in the other. The ticket agent said that unfortunately his reservation had been cleared and his seat given away. She politely and kindly told him that she would do everything she could to get him a seat on a later flight.

Well, he went ballistic. Everyone in the terminal could hear his frustration. He had an important meeting in Los Angeles, and he had to get there. I couldn't help but feel for him because I've been in similar situations where I couldn't afford to miss a flight, but everybody felt sorry for the ticket agent, especially when in his tirade he yelled out that he wanted to see a supervisor.

Suddenly, a woman who appeared to be in her seventies walked up to the man and said that she wasn't in a hurry and that she would be happy to give him her seat. As you can imagine, the man stopped right in his tracks. It almost looked as if he was about to cry. He apologized to her, to the ticket agent, and to everyone around for his behavior and thanked the woman for being an angel in his life. He boarded the flight smiling, relieved, and much wiser! What a blessing for the lovely woman, too. The man never knew it, of course, but the airline got her on another flight just three hours later and also gave her a free, first-class, round-trip ticket to any destination served by the company. So she was truly twice blessed.

As Mother Teresa once said, "Spread your love everywhere you go." Walk the path of love and kindness, and joy will be your constant companion.

LET YOUR HEART-LIGHT SHINE

Sometimes we get so caught up in our responsibilities and commitments to family, friends, work, and doing what's expected of us that there is little left to give to others, let alone ourselves. In times like this, we need to step outside the ordinaryand enter into the realm of the extraordinary and magnificent. With willingness and a little effort, you can create miracles in your life and the lives of others. You can become an angel, transforming the lives of others simply by giving with love.

Something as simple as reaching out with a kind act or word of praise or appreciation can mean so much to others, but so often we seem to assume that others have it all together and don't need our kindness. Wouldn't it be better to move beyond our assumptions and offer the kind of thoughtfulness we would appreciate receiving—a compliment, a smile, a hug, a pat on the shoulder, a note of thanks, or just a question that shows concern?Even if your kind gesture goes unnoticed or is refused, it doesn't matter, because in giving to another, you give to yourself.

If you need a place to start, begin by smiling. Everyone can do it. If you're not used to smiling, practice in the mirror by pulling up on the corners of your mouth! Smiling is so simple and yet so effective. Learn to smile sincerely, from your heart. Did you know that it takes more muscular effort to frown than it does to smile? Smile at family and friends, at strangers, at everyone you meet or pass during the day today. Do you realize how many lives you can touch simply by smiling? When you give a smile to one person, he or she catches the good feeling and smiles at another person, and so on, until your smile has indirectly affected the lives of several thousand people in one day. Smile at everyone today and set off a wave of good feeling.

Or how about writing a note of thanks or appreciation? You don't need a special occasion to send a card or note to someone. You may think you're too busy to write something on paper, but it really doesn't take much time. It may even be quicker than the telephone. I love to send cards and letters and am very faithful to this practice, as most of my close friends will attest. Sometimes I'll go to a card store and purchase several dozen cards to have on hand. It's a very harmless addiction! Isn't it fun to receive a card from a friend for no reason at all?

Random acts of kindness that involve money can be satisfying, too. Last week a friend and I were having dinner at a local restaurant. It was early evening and the restaurant wasn't busy, so we had the opportunity to visit with our waitress. We found out that she was a single mom in her early twenties with two children, and that she was putting herself through college by working at two jobs just to make ends meet. In spite of all her challenges, she was sanguine and a joy to be around. When we got our bill, my friend and I decided to do something special, just because we could. Even though the bill was under $30, we left a $100 tip. What a great feeling to see the look on our waitress's face when she discovered her good fortune and rich blessing!

Treat a friend to a meal or a cup of tea.

Sometimes the kindest gestures may not even be noticed. When I walk down the street, I love to put coins in parking meters if I see any that have expired. The drivers of the cars may never know, but it makes me feel good that I may have spared them a parking ticket. From time to time I put a few dollars in an envelope and send it anonymously to someone I know is in need. It takes so little to do so much.

Sometimes gestures are very much noticed. When I was in Oregon not long ago, my wonderful friend Helen accompanied me to a radio station, where I did an interview from 11 p.m. to midnight. After the interview was over, the radio station closed and everyone left. Helen and I walked to my car, only to discover that it wouldn't start. I lifted the hood to see if anything looked out of the ordinary. Helen reminded me that we were not in the best area of town and blocks from a telephone. It was cold and beginning to rain. I told Helen that we needed to imagine and affirm that an angel would help us out of this dilemma.

As we were getting back into the car to see if an angel would start the engine, a cab drove by. The driver stopped and asked if we needed any help. Helen whispered to me to have faith, even though he didn't look like the angel she had imagined. I agreed. The cabdriver looked under the hood and immediately checked the battery. It was out of water. He had a jug of water in his cab and filled the reservoirs. He also told us an interesting story. He had just dropped off a passenger several blocks away and was heading home, since his shift was over. Something inside him guided him to take a totally different route that evening, one he had never taken before. He thought it was odd but did it anyway. That's when he saw Helen and me looking under the hood and wondered if we needed help. When we told him that he was the angel we had imagined, his delighted smile warmed our hearts. He followed us in his cab all the way back to my home to make sure the car didn't stall, then said good-bye.

That's not the end of the story. The next day I found a book about angels left "anonymously" on my doorstep. But Helen and I both knew who left it. Were these random acts of kindness, or were they specifically the work of angels? I don't believe it matters, because they blessed us, and they blessed our "angelic" cabdriver.

William Penn described well the act of kindness when he wrote, "If there is any kindness I can show, or any good thing

I can do to any fellow being, let me do it now, and not deter or neglect it, as I shall not pass this way again."

REACH OUT AND TOUCH SOMEONE

In his inspiring book *Joy Is My Compass*, Alan Cohen writes that "the difference between a saint and a sourpuss is that the sourpuss sees his daily interactions as a nuisance, while the saint finds a continuous stream of opportunities to celebrate. One finds intruders, the other angels. At any given moment we have the power to choose what we will be and what we will see. Each of us has the capacity to find holiness or attack all about us." By our intentions and through our attitudes we can choose to see heaven or hell. Choosing heaven has so many advantages.

A few years ago, a friend and I went to see a play in Los Angeles. When it was over, we decided to get something to eat at a cafe down the street. It was late and few people were in the restaurant. After a while I noticed a ragged woman, probably in her mid-fifties, who obviously didn't feel good about herself. The waitress told us that she came in every Saturday evening at the same time. While I was talking with my friend, I couldn't help but notice the woman's appearance. Her clothes were dirty, her hair was matted and greasy, and she carried a backpack as her purse. I could sense her sadness and loneliness and was keenly aware of my desire to reach out to her, but I didn't really know what to do.

My friend had to leave, but I decided to stay. I went over to the woman's table, touched her hand, and asked her to keep me company while I finished my meal. At that point she started to cry, and I thought to myself, "Susan, you certainly misread your inner signals this time." As I sat down to try and mend the situation, the woman, Gloria, told me I was the first person to approach her with genuine warmth and caring in months! We talked for an hour, and then she invited me to her apartment a couple of blocks away. In her cramped, disheveled one-room apartment I listened through the night to her life story.

I found out that Gloria hadn't worked for months and that she had no family and rarely had visitors. As she spoke of her love for children, I remembered a telephone call I had received two weeks before. A friend who owns a day care center had called, asking me if I could recommend someone for an opening as a teacher's aide. I will never forget the sparkle in Gloria's eyes when I told her the details of this possible job.

It was now eight o'clock in the morning. I suggested she take a shower, and then we could return to the coffee shop for breakfast. I also called the day care center owner. The position was still open, and I arranged for Gloria to have an interview later that day. In the meantime, I helped Gloria curl her hair, showed her how to apply some makeup, and helped her pick out a clean dress to wear for the interview. It was wonderful to see her transform before my eyes. Gloria got the job and began work the next week.

After several weeks, I paid a surprise visit to Gloria at the center. I could hardly believe my eyes. She looked ten years younger and was aglow with enthusiasm. The children all loved her, and so did the center's owner. She invited me to her apartment for dinner that evening. I didn't recognize her home, either. She had cleaned and painted every inch and even had a couple of plants on her dresser. I was so touched. Gloria was radiantly alive and happy, as she was meant to be.

From this experience I truly learned the value of reaching out to someone, even though we have no guarantee of the outcome. I believe we have to try to live that way—person to person, heart to heart. Life is not a spectator sport. Participate in the adventure of living. You cannot induce positive change in someone by doing for them what they can and should do for themselves, but you can be a catalyst for change. With love in your heart and a willingness to take risks and be vulnerable, you'll do all right.

THE HEALTH BENEFITS OF SMALL PLEASURES

Being kind and gentle begins with how we treat ourselves. Too many of us excel at being tough on ourselves. We beat ourselves up when we make a mistake, choose incorrectly, or repeat the past. Try being kind and understanding with yourself. Be especially kind to yourself if you behave in a way that you dislike. Always talk kindly to yourself, and be patient when you find it difficult to be a "holy" person. Forgive yourself, and when you do not act as you would like, use your actions to remind you where you are and where you want to be. Be your own best friend. This is the most important step on the path to joy and health.

A clinical study uncovered a surprising physical benefit from working small joys into our day-to-day schedule: It can help give our immune system a boost. Researchers in the department of psychiatry at State University of New York at Stony Brook asked one hundred volunteers to fill out an evaluation of daily ups and downs. They then compared this information with antibody activity in the participants' saliva, a test that indicates immune system fluctuations. They found that the stress of a negative event weakens the immune system on the day it occurs, but a positive event can strengthen the immune system for two days or more.

"In other words, positive daily events help immune function more than upsetting events hurt it," says Arthur Stone, PhD, the psychologist who conducted the study. Among the everyday events that boosted subjects' immune systems: pursuing leisure activities, such as gardening or walking in nature, and spending time on a favorite hobby or special interest. Take time to be kind to yourself with life-affirming pleasures and activities.

THE HEALTH BENEFITS OF LOVE AND KINDNESS

Often in today's society we are tempted to put our selfish interests first, before loyalty or integrity or commitment to higher values. Since what emanates from us will come back to us at some point, this is ultimately not a winning attitude. We must do what is right for the sake of doing what is right. True friendship can be one of the rewards. The love shared between two people is the most precious gift we have. I love what Sir Hugh Walpole said: "The most wonderful of all things in life, I believe, is the discovery of another human being with whom one's relationship has a glowing depth, beauty, and joy as the years increase. This inner progression of love between two human beings is a most marvelous thing, it cannot be found by looking for it or by passionately wishing for it. It is a sort of divine accident."

This sentiment reminds me of my beautiful friend, Molly. Well into her seventies when I met her, she certainly knew how to celebrate life and how to be kind and loving—it was evident in her many friendships. The occasions we spent visiting together will always be special to me. A vibrant, alive, and positive woman, Molly spent her days swimming, walking, doing yoga, and volunteering at the UCLA hospital. When she was diagnosed with terminal cancer, the shocking news darkened her sunny disposition for the first three days. Then she adjusted to it and decided to make the most of whatever time she had left. She continued her routine and seemed as radiantly alive and cheerful as ever.

In the last month of her life, Molly was a patient in the hospital where she had volunteered for so long. I was away on a lengthy speaking tour, and when I returned I immediately went to visit her.

I wasn't prepared for what I saw. During my absence she had lost nearly half her body weight, all her teeth, and most of her color, but—astonishingly—not her cheerful attitude. Although she was physically unrecognizable, her spirit shone through when she said, "Sunny, I know I've looked better. Let's see if you can perform your magic and fix me up." I brushed her hair, washed her face, and applied a drop of her favorite perfume. Although she could barely move and had difficulty speaking, she still told me a couple of jokes. She also spoke with great appreciation about the flowers in her room and the birds singing to her from the tree outside her window.

She then asked me to lie down next to her, because she needed to talk and she didn't think she had much time. In that final hour she spoke to me about the light and colors she saw and about the peace and joy she felt. She was ready to cross over to the other side and was actually eager to make her transition. Just before she died she said to me, "Life is meant to be joyful. Don't ever get too serious about life. Laugh every day and live each day as though it were your last. Continue to find ways to give love to others like you have always done with me. Follow your heart and let the beauty of life into your spirit." And then she passed on.

My experiences with Molly taught me so many precious and invaluable life lessons that have taken up permanent residence in my heart, like this one:

One of the greatest hungers of every human heart is to feel understood.

Molly also reminded me that we must embrace all of life and live every day as though we were born anew. Erich Fromm said, "Living is the process of continuous rebirth. The tragedy in the life of most of us is that we die before we are fully born."

My experiences with Molly also make me think of something Elisabeth Kübler-Ross said in her book *Death: The Final Stage of Growth*. "What is important is to realize that whether we understand fully who we are or what will happen when we die, it's our purpose to grow as human beings, to look within ourselves, to find and build upon that source of peace and understanding and strength that is our individual self. And then to reach out to others with love and acceptance and patient guidance in the hope of what we may become together."

SHOWING KINDNESS DAY TO DAY

Practice makes us better at recognizing those daily opportunities to show kindness toward ourselves and others. If you're looking for new ideas, here are some to add to your list:

- Go to your local shelter and adopt a pet.
- Offer a ride to a friend who can't get around.
- Volunteer at your local library.
- Pick up some trash as you walk down the sidewalk.
- Ask your friends and coworkers to tell you their stories of random acts of kindness. Have a party just for that purpose.
- Give another person your parking spot, or let another driver get in front of you if they want. Wave and smile at them, too!
- Surprise a forgotten friend or relative with a phone call.
- Give a present to an underprivileged boy or girl, or to someone you know, for no reason at all.
- Take the clothes you haven't worn in a year to a homeless shelter. Organize neighbors on your block to do the same.
- Wave hello to pedestrians when you're in your car, even if you don't know them. It will lift their spirits, as well as yours.
- Let the person behind you in line at the grocery or hardware store go in front of you. Pay for their purchases, too, if

you can. If they are hesitant, just tell them it will make you feel terrific.

- When you're in line for a movie, anonymously pay for the ticket of someone behind you in line. Watch their face when they receive the news.
- Order a gift anonymously for someone you know who needs to be cheered up, or slip a $20 bill into the pocket or purse of a needy friend or stranger.
- If you drive on a toll bridge, pay for the next few cars after yours.
- Laugh out loud and smile often. Even when you're not in the mood to smile, do it. It will lift everybody's spirits.
- If you know someone who's having a difficult day, do something special for them without telling them you did it.
- Tell your family and friends often how much you appreciate them and how blessed you are to have their presence in your life.
- Tell your boss or employees the same things. Everyone wants and needs to feel appreciated.
- If you have children, get them to go through their toys and select some to give to less fortunate kids. Let your children go with you to take the toys someplace they will be appreciated.
- Plant a tree or flowers in your neighbor's yard or somewhere they are needed—with permission, of course!
- Take a beautiful plant to your local nursing home, fire station, hospital, police station, or doctor's office.
- Make sandwiches, drive by a city park, and give them to homeless people
- Leave a flower anonymously on someone's windshield.
- Look in the mirror every day and tell yourself how beautiful and wonderful you are.
- Compliment others whenever you can.
- If you see someone who appears stressed or unhappy, visualize them surrounded by Light and Love.
- Be loving and kind to yourself every day, knowing that you deserve to live a happy, joy-filled, wonderful life.

I slept and dreamt that life was joy.
I awoke and saw that life was service.
I acted and behold service was joy.
—RABINDRANATH TAGORE

It isn't enough to talk about peace. One must believe in it. And it isn't
enough to believe in it. One must work at it.
—ELEANOR ROOSEVELT

CHAPTER 3

Celebrate the Child in You

I CHOOSE TO APPROACH LIFE AS
A PLAYFUL ADVENTURE

*This ability to see, experience, and accept the new is one of our
saving characteristics. If we accept the new with joy and wonder,
we can move gracefully into each tomorrow. More often than not,
the children shall lead us.*
—LEO BUSCAGLIA

*I have great hope for tomorrow. And my hope lies in the following three
things: truth, youth, and love.*
—BUCKMINSTER FULLER

A few years ago I decided to give a party in my front yard for
several neighborhood children, who ranged in age from three to
six. Just before the party was to begin, I received an upsetting telephone call. The caller was a close friend, and we were not seeing
eye-to-eye on something important to both of us. What started
out calmly ended in raised voices and feelings of frustration.

I had to go back outside to greet my young guests as they
arrived. The toys, decorations, and snacks were ready, but I felt
like calling the whole thing off. I'm so glad I didn't. That day
became one of the most memorable days of my life. In no time at
all, I had forgotten about my telephone conversation and become
totally involved with the children, allowing myself to become a
child again, too.

As we played together, I realized that children instinctively
understand the secret of living fully. They are totally fascinated
by their world and unmindful of the problems of yesterday or
tomorrow. They give themselves the freedom to embrace life with

passion, to be totally absorbed in the present, and to welcome the unfamiliar and out-of-the-ordinary. Their moments appear to be almost magical.

I have always had a great fondness for children. While I was still living with my family, during high school and my first year at UCLA, the neighbors' children would often come to my home to see if I could come out and play. I could rarely resist. I remember vividly the games we would play, the endless laughter, the many moments when we were silly and goofy. Those times will always hold a special place in my heart. When was the last time you played hide-and-go-seek with some children, or tag, or pin the tail on the donkey? Can you remember what you loved to do when you were a child? I remember riding my bike, pretending it was a magnificent white stallion with wings, and I can still feel the wind rushing through my hair as we "galloped" swiftly along!

Even today, some of my best times are spent with children. I can often be found at a local park, playground, or beach with a group of small friends, playing ball, swinging, running, feeding birds, or just laughing a lot. Children never ask, but adults have asked me numerous times during my life why I don't act my age. As long as I continue to hear that, I figure I must be doing just fine. Charles Dickens wrote, "To the young at heart, everything is fun."

CHILDLIKE VERSUS CHILDISH

You don't have to give up being an adult in order to become more childlike. There is a big difference, however, between being childlike and being childish. To be childish means either to be a child and act like one, which is perfectly normal, or to be an adult and act like a child in ways that indicate your growth and maturity were somehow impeded and that you have been stagnated and callow ever since. To be childlike means to be innocent of strange, authoritarian ideas of what adulthood ought to be; to be trusting and straightforward; and to be more concerned with living life than with how you look to others. It is not necessary to be infantile or the least bit irresponsible or unaccountable. The fully integrated person incorporates a harmonious blend of adult and child.

If, as I believe, the child in each of us is waiting to come forth and express itself more fully, what keeps us from getting back in touch with it? It's usually our own unwillingness to recognize and accept that child. Often we think, "Now that I'm grown up, I have to act my age."

There is a lovely passage in the Bible (Matthew 19:14): "Let the children come to me, and do not hinder them; for to such belongs the kingdom of heaven." Young children live in their own heaven, no matter what their background, the language they speak, or where they live. Children's celebration of life, passion, and joy is universal.

Once, while I was jogging in a park in Switzerland, I noticed several children playing a game that was new to me. Their parents and nannies were sitting quietly, not talking or paying much attention to the children. The kids were having a fantastic time laughing, running, touching, being silly, and enjoying one another's company. It looked like so much fun. After watching for a few minutes, I felt compelled to join them. Through hand signals I asked if I could play, and an hour later I was exhausted. Although I couldn't speak their language, we laughed a whole lot. There was a special bonding and love, a respect and sharing, that transcended the need for words. Laughter can be so freeing and so uniting at the same time.

The very next day, toward the end of my walk, I saw a boy and girl down on all fours, looking keenly at the ground next to a beautiful flowering tree. I stopped to see what was so captivating. In intermittent English, their mother told me that for nearly thirty minutes the two children had been engrossed in watching some ants as they made their journey from the tree to a scattering of bread crumbs a few feet away. Then and there I got down on my hands and knees, too, and for several precious minutes I joined the children in their adventure, becoming totally involved with them and the ants. It was delightful.

Reflect a moment on your own experiences being around children. What are children like? How do you feel when you are with them? What qualities do they express to you? Before you read on, write down some words that would describe your favorite children. As you read over the list, ask yourself how many of these qualities are part of your personality. Which ones would you like to develop or reawaken?

When I wrote my list, the evening after my neighborhood party, here are some words that came to my mind: Children are

- sanguine
- alert
- eager

- trusting
- persevering
- open

They are also

- energetic
- cheerful
- caring
- playful

- sensitive
- friendly
- inquisitive
- vivacious

They are enthusiastic, playful, expressive, spontaneous, and natural. They laugh a lot and love to act silly and crazy. They are innocently loving and incredibly lovable. Your list may contain other adjectives, but from my perspective, these positive childlike qualities are the guaranteed recipe for living fully. As children grow older, they are strongly influenced by the behavior of their role models and the mores of their society. This influence provides all the more reason for us to model for children a playful, childlike way to be a responsible adult.

LET THE CHILD IN YOU COME OUT TO PLAY

There are all kinds of ways to let the child in you out for a great adventure. I have been known to get my friends involved by renting videos like *Enchanted, Shrek, Finding Nemo, Babe,* or *Eloise at the Plaza.* I invite a few close friends over to watch these movies with me, but I make two requests: to come dressed as a little child, and to bring a favorite toy. When the guests arrive, they are greeted by me and my very special teddy bear, Golden. Ah! Dressing up like this to see a movie may sound silly, but it's a wonderful way to remind ourselves how we felt when everything was new and exciting. Rediscovering the adventure of life is a glorious gift, free and available to everyone. We simply have to recognize and accept the child within us who knows how to be happy, healthy, and creatively alive.

Think about it. Isn't it fun to be around people who can let their inner child come out to play? They are usually upbeat, fully functioning people who haven't forgotten that it is possible to be happy and responsible at the same time, who aren't afraid of what others think, and who can occasionally become totally immersed in fantasy, just as they did when they were children.

You may think there's no way you can act like a child. You have a job with many responsibilities, bills to pay, and many problems and frustrations to deal with. But understand that children have problems and frustrations, too. They have tests in school, difficulties with friends, and problems with parents, yet they bring a different attitude to life's situations. Children handle things as they come up, without taking life so seriously. Young people can often show great wisdom and resilience. You don't have to stop acting like an adult— just try to let the inner child influence the adult's thoughts and feelings. That's the key to celebrating life.

One way to achieve this blend is to spend time around children. Watch them. Play with them. Get involved. Throw yourself into their activities. Pretend you are a child again. If you haven't any children of your own, find a way to be with children on a regular basis. You can always volunteer somewhere: as a Big Sister or Big Brother, with the Boy or Girl Scouts, in a school as a teacher's aide or in the pediatric ward of a nearby hospital. I know you will find it worthwhile. Children have a way of revealing us to ourselves, if we can be open with them. They are like mirrors, showing us many valuable lessons about living.

BE ALL THAT YOU CAN BE

My mom always used to say to me that "the more you love, the more you're loved and the lovelier you are." Love is who we are, and our Heart-Light's pilot light is always on, shining through the darkness of insecurities, low self-esteem, lack of confidence, and shyness. But with a little courage and willingness to let our Heart-Light shine, we can inspire others to do the same. In other words, be your most radiant, vibrant Self and you'll attract the same radiance back to you. Being all that we can be means being authentic, sensitive, vulnerable, and willing to express our feelings. When we're being who we are, we don't wear masks, we have no pretenses, and we are ingenuous. Children exhibit these qualities when they meet a new friend. Even though they might start out with some timidity and shyness, when it feels right (and for children it almost always does), they relate as though they were long-time friends.

At my party, three of the children were new to the neighborhood and didn't know anyone. But within the first few minutes, they were all getting along like best buddies, sharing toys and food with no displays of cupidity or pugnacity.

Compare this approach with your own feelings and behavior when you meet someone new. How do you respond? How long is your initial period of shyness? Are you likely to feel reserved or suspicious? If you are, perhaps these feelings are related to how you feel about yourself. Do you attempt to curry favor or maybe display reticence? The ability to trust lies in your mind and is expressed through your attitude. Our thoughts and feelings about ourselves have a great influence on our circumstances. What you believe to be true about yourself and about your world will be duplicated in all your life experiences.

The next time you meet a new person, be aware of your reactions. Notice if you are being cool or keeping the person at arm's length with small talk. See if you are wondering what this person is after. Are you feeling a little uncomfortable, perhaps, uncertain about where this new encounter might be headed? Take your cue from kids, who can have a great time together and enjoy the present moment, even if they know they may never see each other again. Set right out to find this new person's funny bone, or find some other way to disarm or put him or her at ease. When you show that you accept and respect someone, their barriers immediately begin to drop. If you let your childlike trust take over and feel positive about being able to relate to anyone who comes along, your very attitude of certainty will see you through.

Make a point of meeting someone new this week. Make a habit of introducing yourself to people you don't know, even if it feels funny at first. This habit will help shake off your inhibitions about talking to strangers. Trust new friends and yourself to make the best of the situation. Find out what it is you have in common. The more you do this, the more you'll discover, as I have, that what we have in common with one another far outweighs our differences. Furthermore, it's the differences that make friendships stimulating and exciting.

Allow your inner child to show you how to make new friends, how to be a friend, and how to start living with élan. The child in you knows how to deal with everyone and every situation with perfect aplomb. Best of all, the child is eager to give love and affection.

If you care for your family and friends, never hesitate to let them know. You don't have to wait for birthdays and anniversaries. Make every day Valentine's Day. If you have a difficult time expressing your feelings verbally, send a card, offer a hug or a pat, or give someone flowers. When my mom was alive, we talked often, and when we finished talking we always ended by telling each other, "I love you." That meant so much to me. Remember, too, that even though a loving message might not be received or acknowledged the way you would wish, it's still worth sending. Live today as though it were your last day. Be the friend or loved one you would appreciate having.

GIVE FANTASY ITS WINGS AND FLY

Another way to live fully is through fantasy or creative daydreaming. Remember how, when you were a child, your bedroom could be a world unto itself? Sometimes it was a fortress, perhaps, and other times it was another planet. Remember when you dressed up in costumes or when you pretended you were a grocer, doctor, pilot, athlete, actor, singer, or ballet dancer? For adults as well as children, creative daydreaming provides a practical escape from the pressures of everyday living. It eliminates boredom and enhances creativity. Dreaming does more than just that, in fact—it creates our reality. All of our present realities started with thoughts, dreams, and visualization. Dreams and goals give our thoughts a positive direction. Too many of us waste time thinking about all the negative elements around us or about how others should change to meet our expectations. When we are focusing on what we want and where we are headed, we can't be worrying about what we don't want or don't have. Remember, what we think about consistently, we draw into our lives.

This maxim was never more apparent to me than it was several years ago on a ski trip to Sun Valley with the UCLA Ski Club. The package included a flight to a city in Idaho, where the group was to catch a bus for the long ride to Sun Valley. I bought my ticket early and looked forward to the trip for weeks. On the day of departure, my mom dropped me off at the airport. I checked in, got my seat assignment, and boarded the plane. I was puzzled at not seeing any of my friends who were also scheduled to be on the trip, but figured they must be sitting toward the back. After the plane landed, I still didn't see any of my friends at the baggage claim area. Bewildered and concerned, I headed for the outdoor curb where, according to my ski information packet, the buses would be waiting. I found no friends or buses anywhere! I called the bus company to find out why the buses were late. The person on the other end of the line sounded amused as he said: "The buses will be there on time—tomorrow." Tomorrow?!

I pride myself on being an organized, efficient, and accountable person, so you can imagine my astonishment. How was it that I had marked the day on my calendar, talked with my friends about the upcoming ski trip without discovering the erroneous date, and encountered no problems at the airport when the ticket

I presented was dated for the following day? Bemused as well as nonplussed, I decided to make the best of it. I made a reservation at a nearby hotel with a sauna, gym, and salad bar. After the taxi dropped me off, I called my mom and we had a good laugh about my oversight. I then bundled up in sweats and ski hat and went out for a jog in the freshly fallen snow.

After a while, I came across an inviting health food store. It had a small restaurant and I decided to get some soup. As I waited for the waitress to take my order, I became aware of an elderly man sitting a few tables away. He was staring at me with a weird expression on his face, which made me feel very uncomfortable. As I looked back at him, his stare changed from inquisitiveness to pure shock. I noticed his wife asking him if he was okay. Pointing toward me, he continued to stare while his wife turned in my direction. Then, apprehensively, the man stood up and came to my table. With noticeable difficulty in forming his words, he asked, "Are you Susan Smith Jones?" I couldn't believe someone there had recognized me, especially under my layers of clothing and hat. When I answered, he and his wife gasped.

It turned out that one week before, this man had sat in the very same health food store reading an article I had written about creative visualization and the importance of positive daydreaming. I wrote about how, if you believe enough, you can use visualization and creative thoughts to create any reality you choose. After reading this article, which included a photograph of me, the man said to his wife how much he would like to meet and talk with me. His wife skeptically suggested that he visualize meeting me, which is exactly what he had been doing during the past week. In most of his daydreams he focused on sitting with me and asking me all his personal health questions, since he was aware that I worked as a holistic health and lifestyle coach.

Neither the man nor his wife will ever again question the validity and power of creative visualization, nor will I. This was far beyond mere coincidence. We talked for several hours and shared many stories, and I answered a barrage of health questions. The man was contemplating bypass surgery at his doctor's recommendation. I clearly outlined for him the wellness lifestyle program described in my books and my audio programs *Choose to Live Peacefully* and *Wired to Meditate*. I wrote out the heart-friendly diet and suggested he start it immediately, especially in light of the fact that his doctor had told him his diet wouldn't make any difference. (As you can imagine, I suggested that he seek out another doctor with nutrition knowledge.) I also encouraged him to begin a program of walking, meditation, and stretching as well as sleeping more and doing positive visualizations about his health. As a result of my suggestions and his willingness to embrace a new holistic health program, his surgery was canceled. His doctor was astonished at the reversal of his coronary heart disease.

Thanks to this episode and countless others, I've come to realize that there is an unfathomable yet perfectly recognizable Divine Order to our universe. It's ever-present, irrepressible, and always working in alignment with what we need for our highest good and spiritual unfolding and growth. I've learned not to analyze or question it anymore. I continue to live in awe of this alignment and the magnificent adventure life continually is. It was Helen Keller who wrote: "Life is either a daring adventure or nothing. To keep our faces toward change and behave like free spirits in the presence of fate is strength undefeatable."

Make friends with your fantasies. Always imagine and think about what you want in life and, at the same time, let go of all thoughts of what you don't want. Let your imagination work for you and not against you. (I write about visualization and coincidence in greater detail in Chapter 8.) Again, turn to children as models. Children have the ability not to put limits on their thinking and dreaming. Anything is possible for those who believe, and children understand this better than anyone. They possess limitless dreams and goals, and express their aspirations easily. If you are a parent or otherwise have children in your life, encourage them to fantasize and to share their dreams with you, so that they can carry the gift of creative daydreaming into their adult lives.

If you have forgotten your fantasy life, you might try finding some children with whom to laugh and play. Encourage everyone to share their wildest dreams. You will discover how spontaneously creative children can be, and it will rub off on you. Think about some of your dreams and fantasies. Have you ever wanted to go sailing or surfing? How about river rafting or snorkeling? Maybe you've wanted to take a cooking class, paint with watercolors, visit Bali, learn karate, embrace a live-food diet for 30 days, play the banjo, spend a few days completely alone and silent, or camp overnight in the mountains. Whatever your dreams are, make a list. It doesn't matter how crazy or silly these things may seem. You don't need to justify to anyone why you want to do these things. Simply wanting to do something that feeds your heart and soul is reason enough to do it.

Now look over your list. Some things you wrote down will be difficult to do right away, but I'm sure you listed at least one thing that you can do immediately. Do it today. Keep your list of dreams and keep adding to it, as well as crossing off things you've accomplished or about which you've changed your mind.

Things on my list that I've been fortunate enough to carry out include skydiving, hang gliding, a vision quest, motocross, painting, Tai Chi, photography, and camping alone in the mountains. I even tried bungee jumping. Was I scared? You bet! But after the jump, I felt as if there was nothing I couldn't do. The other bonus was that when I jumped, I got a free chiropractic adjustment at the same time. What a thrill! Still on my list are: design and build my dream home; take singing lessons; learn to play the piano well, win the Pulitzer Prize; visit Paris in springtime and Tuscany in the fall; spend a summer each in Italy and France; host my own cooking and healthy living talk show; drive up the California, Oregon, and Washington coast in a hybrid automobile without any agenda or planned schedule; see one of my books reach number one on the *Los Angeles Times* and *New York Times* bestseller lists; climb Mt. Whitney. I'd also love to spend the day with actors Steve Martin, Denzel Washington, Meryl Streep, Rita Wilson and her husband Tom Hanks, director Ron Howard, American investor, industrialist, and philanthropist Warren Buffett, American philanthropist Eli Broad, stylist Tim Gunn, and designer Vera Wang , and Prince William—interview them, watch them work, and enjoy their company—or visit with some of my other favorite role models, like Diane Sawyer, Oprah Winfrey, Bonnie Hunt, Tyra Banks, Rachel Ray, Martha Stewart, Tyra Banks, Rachel Ray, Martha Stewart, Ellen DeGeneres, Barbara Walters, Steven Spielberg, and the Dalai Lama. (Let's just say I'm eclectic.) Which one of these dreams can I do today? I leave it to you to guess! Some of them may take a little longer, but before too long I'll be able to cross them off as completed, too.

LIVING IN THE PRESENT

What is it about children's play that we long for? Children allow themselves to be totally involved in the moment, focused on whatever they are doing right now. Their attention span may not be long, but when they eat, they just eat; when they play, they just play; when they talk, they just talk. They throw themselves wholeheartedly into their activity, without any sense of time or the duration of things. When I was a small child, my family took frequent long trips in the car. Anybody who has taken a long car trip with a small child knows what happened. Usually within ten minutes of leaving home I would ask, "Are we there yet?" followed by "When are we going to be there?" The questions were repeated every few minutes, because "two hours away" doesn't mean anything to children. Their only time is now.

I am not recommending that you forget the past or the future. I believe not just in dreaming but in planning ahead and preparing for the future. Plans have their time and place, but most of the time, remind yourself to be here, now. Be open to the sounds, sights, and feelings of every minute as you experience it. Appreciate life with all of your senses.

Once again, we can turn to children for inspiration. Have you ever noticed that children are willing to try anything at a moment's notice? Even though they may have done the very same thing before, they will express wide-eyed excitement and wonderment. This is because children don't use a yardstick to measure activities or compare the present with the past. They know they've played the game before, or had someone read them the same story just last night, yet it's still as fresh and wonderful as it was the first time.

Often when I'm conducting a workshop in a beautiful setting, I ask the participants to go outside for 15 minutes and saunter around the grounds alone, in silence. I have them practice being totally absorbed in what they can see, smell, taste, feel, and hear. To be with nature, letting its beauty into your awareness, is wonderful. What I have discovered in taking this kind of walk (and I do this at least once a week) is that I feel a subtle, gentle communion with nature. Each time the senses are engaged by different things, and everyone who tries it finds something new, as if walking outside were a totally new experience.

When was the last time you walked past a school playground when the children were playing? Did you notice how totally involved they are, oblivious to past annoyances and future problems? Children let their spontaneity run free. One moment they may be completely absorbed in a certain game and then, minutes later, they will change games and be just as completely absorbed in a new activity.

If you are like many people, your schedule is tightly planned. It's entirely appropriate, if you have goals, to make plans and be disciplined with your time. But if you are too rigid, if your schedule is too strict, it will be difficult for your inner child to come out and enjoy life. Plato's words, "Life must be lived as play," are important to keep in mind No matter how scheduled or unscheduled your life is at present, block out a specific time each day that's free from any scheduled activity. Then, when the time rolls around, see what you feel like doing. How about daydreaming, writing a letter, going to the park, or taking a ride on your bike? Just ride, and see where you end up. See what moves you at the moment. As you tune in more to the child in you, it will show you more and more how you can thoroughly enjoy each day and how being more spontaneous will add a new dimension to your life.

"Life must be lived as play." —Plato

If your present moment is obscured by "should have," or "if only," or "maybe tomorrow," try the following exercise: Write down some of your self-limiting thoughts, beliefs, and habits—

anything that keeps you from doing all that you can do and being all that you can be right now. Take your time. Look deeply within yourself, and include as many of your current hurdles as you can think of. Then put your list in a brown paper bag. Close the top securely. Breathing deeply and slowly, put the bag in a fireplace or somewhere safe and set it on fire. Watch all of your excess baggage disintegrate before your eyes. Just let it go. And as it disappears, affirm something such as: "I choose to embrace and celebrate my life moment to moment and honor my heart's wishes with resounding joy and gratitude."

DON'T BE AFRAID TO MAKE MISTAKES OR FAIL

Too often we stop ourselves from venturing past our comfort zone for fear of what others will think or for fear of failure. Failure is only a word. It has no power other than what we give it. Children haven't yet learned the adult meaning of the word failure, and thus they are eager to take risks most of the time. They intuitively know that to risk is to learn and grow. Have you ever watched a child learning to ride a bike—falling, getting up, and starting over again and again, no matter how many times it takes? The child isn't trying to prove anything to anyone else and isn't afraid of failing repeatedly in order to reach a goal. What is failure, anyway? Just a delay in results and a way of seeing which choices worked for you and which didn't.

Fear of making a mistake or looking foolish is just as great a deterrent to living fully as is fear of failure. At my children's party, we played a game that was all about letting go of self-consciousness. It involved laying a large sheet of plastic on the grassy slope. Then we turned on the hose and ran water over the plastic sheet. We ran and slid over it, twisting, spinning, and getting entangled with one another. There was no way to do it "right," and nobody cared the least bit how foolish he or she looked. It was great fun even though it was easy to slip and fall, as we all did. We had a wonderful time enjoying the moment. Be more concerned with your integrity and experience of living than with what others might think.

ACCEPT THE WORLD AS IT IS

In adulthood we face many conditions that we wish were different, from natural disasters, acts of terrorism, world hunger, environmental pollution, and crime and drug problems to our state of health or looks. Many times, no matter what we do, things don't seem to change fast enough. The key is to get involved in change and at the same time try to keep a child's appreciation of what the present situation may offer. Children don't resist life. They are amazingly accepting and able to take things as they come and make the most of them.

Think of the weather—a natural phenomenon that we clearly cannot control. Let's say it's early morning and we adults have just awakened to discover that it snowed heavily last night. The driveway is full of snow and the roads are a mess. We start to fret and bemoan our fate, dreading the drive to work. Even if we choose to stay home, we are already convinced that the day is wasted. But the children? They haven't been this excited in days. Either they will get to walk through the snow on the way to school or, if they stay home, they'll be able to play all day in this winter wonderland. What heaven!

I remember a few years ago a friend of mine had plans to play tennis, but his plans were thwarted when Mother Nature decided to bless my community in West Los Angeles with some much-needed rain. Instead of finding a way to celebrate the blessing, he sulked around his house all day, angry at the weather. What a waste of precious, sacred time! Your life is just a matter of attitude. Make whatever is going on in your life at the moment okay. Accept what is and what can't be changed, and make the best of it.

Accepting what is includes accepting the way we feel. It's so important to be in touch with your emotions, express them, complete them, and then let them go. Babies do this so marvelously. Think back to the last time you saw a baby really frustrated. (For some of you, it might be within the past few minutes!) A baby will cry his or her heart out and clearly express his vexation. The baby isn't wondering if it's all right to be crying, or feeling guilty or embarrassed for doing so. The baby just cries, then lets it go. Similarly, if a baby is angry, he or she will let you know immediately and then let it go, without holding onto anger or resentment. Babies express themselves fully, then move on. What delightful teachers and what a perfect demonstration of the positive use of energy they are!

It occurs to me that all the magical qualities I appreciate so much in children are also shared by animals. Perhaps that's why I've always been a great lover of animals, especially dogs, cats, birds, and horses. The more I pay attention to how children and animals experience and embrace life, and the more I release my fears about being rejected and feeling uncertain, the better life becomes for me and for the people around me, because I become softer and kinder.

At times, I have come to realize, there's a controlling self within me that can be demanding, perfectionist, and judgmental. Life is far better for me and for those around me when I am able to replace that self with a more accepting, gentle me. When I can forgive and forget, when I can say and feel that whatever happens is all right—when I can take people in my arms or just spiritually embrace them and discover that we are each special, inimitable, and wondrous—then life becomes a great river that will flow no matter what I do. I can flow with it and live in peace, or I can slip back into old patterns and live in frustration, fighting against the current. The river doesn't care what I do. It only makes a difference to me and to those around me. The choice is mine.

For me, the inner child's lesson of accepting and making the most of things is one of the most precious. My efforts to respond to life and to the people I know in a healthy way is not a change I made once and no longer worry about. It is an ongoing venture to be more soft and flexible, to give myself permission to enjoy who I am and what I do and to feel free to laugh, tease, and relax in spontaneous, undemanding ways. When I am successful in allowing those things to happen, my life is better for me and far better for the people around me.

LAUGH AND BE A LITTLE SILLY

When was the last time you really laughed? If you can't remember, you had better read this carefully, because your life might depend on it. Laughter is the lubricant of life, the elixir that enables you to experience the fullness and joy of life. Laugh! Do it often, every day!

Last weekend I was the keynote speaker for a major health fair. My attire included a long, flowing, colorful, flowered skirt and a periwinkle top. I felt happy just looking at all the colors, though I kept thinking how nice it would have been to have green in either the top or skirt. For the past couple of years, green has been my favorite color.

Just before leaving I made a nutritious smoothie for the road. It included romaine lettuce leaves, some spinach leaves, water, and a Bosc pear—all totally green in color. After the greens were blended, I removed the lid to sprinkle in some powdered cinnamon and, because I was in a hurry and not totally mindful of what I was doing, inadvertently forgot to put the top on the blender before starting it up again. You guessed it! Within seconds, my skirt and top had turned entirely green, as had my hair, the kitchen cupboards, the floor, and the ceiling. All I could do was laugh. I ran to the mirror and laughed so hard that my eyes teared up. In the big scheme of things, my mishap was not a big deal, and I had a great story to tell at the health fair.

You've had experiences like this, haven't you? Isn't it better to laugh and let go than to stress ourselves out over these silly and inconsequential events?

If you're not up for laughing, you can practice smiling. Smiling is great for firming your facial muscles; it makes you feel better; it makes people wonder what you've been up to; it's a small curve that sets many things straight; it confuses an approaching frown; and it's the shortest distance between two people.

It takes practice, but it's so important not to take ourselves or life too seriously. Being able to laugh at yourself and the incongruities of everyday situations is the best way to quell stress and to enjoy life.

Remembered laughter can be potent, too, when things are looking gloomy. I can always look back on the day I took my car to a local automatic car wash. I came back outside after paying and noticed that my car was parked separately from all the others. A few other car owners and most of the car wash employees were standing around my car, some looking shocked, some gesturing wildly, and some laughing. At first I thought they were admiring my good-looking automobile, but as I got closer I saw what all the excitement was about—I had forgotten to close the sun roof and there was a lake inside my car! Sheepishly I opened the car door, and out rushed the water. Suddenly it struck me how funny this all was, and I began laughing so hard my stomach hurt and tears rolled down my face. The car did dry out, though it took days and days. It would have done me no good to get upset, and besides, I ended up driving a car with the cleanest interior for miles around. If you have ever wondered what will happen if your sun roof is left open at the car wash, now you know—and you can laugh about it without living through it.

Children are once again our teachers here. They intuitively realize that happiness is a choice—an attitude they create. That's why children often act silly and crazy, making and telling jokes. They know how to see the humor in things, and humor is one of the most important components of wellness.

Laughter and humor really can help make the difference between life and death. In one of my favorite books, *Man's Search for Meaning*, Victor E. Frankl tells the story of his experiences in the Nazi concentration camps and discusses the importance of humor to well being. Yes, humor about being imprisoned: "Humor was another of the soul's weapons in the fight for self-preservation. It is well known that humor, more than anything else in the human make-up, can afford an aloofness and ability to rise above any situation, even if only for a few seconds."

No matter how difficult your circumstances—perhaps particularly in difficult ones—learn to laugh, especially at yourself, and keep on laughing your way through life. Give yourself permission to have fun and be a little giddy.

Every once in a while, a few friends and I go on an adventure I created called a Surprise Hike. Our group starts out on some trail in the local Santa Monica Mountains. Every time we come to a fork in the path, one hiker gets to decide where we go next—straight, right turn, left turn, or about-face. We never know where the journey will take us. It's all a surprise. The person who chooses the direction for a particular portion must also pick a surprise adventure for that part of the trail, which can be just about anything. Some of the things I've suggested are petting a lizard, talking to a rabbit, singing like the birds, dancing with a tree, imitating a deer, or conversing with a pebble that speaks to you. Crazy, you say? Perhaps. But these simple acts help us to focus our attention on the precious present and become more mindful of the beauty, sacredness, and miracles of Nature all around us.

I celebrate four special times each year, at the change of seasons. On these four high-energy days I do special things such as lighting candles and buying flowers reflecting the season's colors. I dance and sing for the sun and moon. I make special gifts, which I offer to Mother Nature. I also celebrate the full and new moons. Sure, I've had more than a few people tell me I'm definitely crazy. I take the remark as a compliment, and I celebrate it. It gives me enormous leeway to be childlike and happy.

Each day, do something a little crazy. Write a silly note and hide it in a family member's shoe or pocket so he or she will find it later. Throw snowballs, fly a kite, skip pebbles over the water, kiss a flower, talk to the animals, greet the sunrise or sunset, go outside in the middle of the night and look for shooting stars, or bring home a birthday cake (carrot, of course) even though it's nobody's birthday. Let go of wondering what other people will think of you. It doesn't matter. What matters is that you enjoy being with yourself and have fun in your own company. When you do, other people will, too.

I was not born to be forced. I will breathe after my own fashion . . .
If a plant cannot live according to its nature, it dies; and so a man.
—HENRY DAVID THOREAU

The story's about you.
—HORACE

Come forth into the light of things,
Let nature be your teacher.
—WILLIAM WORDSWORTH

CHAPTER 4

Resonate to the Music
I CHOOSE THE RICHEST MEDICINE
FOR BODY, MIND, AND SPIRIT

*Use music to elevate your frequency as often as possible, since
it bathes you in shimmering light that deflects negativity.*
—DOREEN VIRTUE

*Develop a deeper friendship with great music, and you will see many areas
of your life begin to open.*
—STEVEN HALPERN

One of the greatest impediments to living fully and celebrating
life is the great stress many of us live with each and every day.
Stress is arguably the major downside to Western-style living at
the beginning of the 21st century. Technological advances have
stepped up life's pace (computers now work in nanoseconds—
billionths of a second!), and created a dizzying abundance of
choices (do we really need hundreds of TV channels?) while at
the same time eliminating jobs through automation. As a result,
a smaller workforce handles a larger workload, often with a cut
in pay. We are likely to be overworked or underemployed, and
in either case over-stimulated. We receive more information in
one day of our lives—thanks to TV, computers, radio, satellites,
etc.—than our ancestors of only a few generations ago could
receive in a thousand days!

The field of psychoneuroimmunology underscores the intricate
relationship between mind and body, stress and disease. Virtually
every month, new studies show the direct effect of psychological

and environmental factors on health. For example, I heard on a CNN News broadcast recently that people under stress are six times more likely to become infected with a cold virus than those who are not stressed. The more stressed we are, the less efficiently our body's immune system works. This cycle of irritation and stress ripples out and has enormous impacts, not the least of them economic. The amount of money lost in the United States alone to stress-related problems in the workforce—absenteeism, illness, and just plain inefficiency on the job—is in the hundreds of billions of dollars per year.

Despite these harsh realities (or perhaps because of them), Americans are increasingly bent on attaining better health, keeping fit, and reducing stress. We seem to have realized that no amount of medical care can take the place of prevention and personal responsibility, and we search for the remedies available to us. So why wait to get sick before you start doing something to make yourself better? Research confirms that stress debilitates and even kills. Inability to handle stress results in addictive disorders, ulcers, migraines, hypertension, obesity, and heart attacks.

The trouble is, most people have not had any training in accurately identifying what relaxation really is. What they think is relaxing is only relaxing compared, say, to being caught in rush hour traffic. Not feeling stressed is good, but it's a long way from being in a meaningful state of relaxation. In a state of deep relaxation, a whole host of beneficial psycho-physiological responses occur that simply do not happen by themselves.

The universally recommended remedy for stress is almost too simple to be believed. Relaxation, just plain "chilling out," when practiced regularly, helps prevent many of today's stress-related diseases and helps us live a healthier life. Relaxation provides:

- Energy
- A more robust immune system
- Enhanced concentration, clarity, and creativity
- Increased ease in falling asleep

BRAINWAVES AND RELAXATION

In 2005, the prestigious *New England Journal of Medicine* announced the results of a major study that concluded that "alternative health care is used by 33 percent of Americans." According to Dr. David Eisenbery of Boston's Beth Israel Hospital and Harvard Medical School, over 60 million Americans now use a variety of alternative therapies instead of, or in addition to, standard Western allopathic medicine. The vast majority seek to achieve more relaxation in their lives.

It is helpful to understand the relationship of alpha and theta brainwave states to relaxation, and the significance of this finding for your personal health and well-being. Once you do, I think you'll agree how important it is to nurture yourself and bring more moments of relaxation into your life.

Scientists have known for a long time that we have different levels of brainwave activity, as measured by different frequencies of electromagnetic wave patterns emanating from the brain. The highest frequency of brainwave activity is exhibited in everyday consciousness and is called the beta range (13–39 cycles per second). Alpha (8–12 cps) and theta (4–7 cps) brainwaves are associated with deep relaxation, meditation, and mental imagery. The result of achieving the lower alpha and theta frequency levels is greater control over your mental state, enhanced creativity, increased productivity, and general feelings of well-being.

Recent discoveries in brain science suggest that each of us has a "Minimum Daily Requirement" of alpha and theta brainwave activity—a requirement of at least 30 minutes every day. Most people do not include enough of these brainwave patterns in their daily schedule, if for no other reason than that they don't know their importance. Yet many behavioral problems are now understood to relate to deficiency of this brainwave activity.

Dr. Eugene Peniston of the V.A. Medical Center in Fort Lyon, Colorado, and Dr. Paul Kulkosky at the University of Southern Colorado, conducted sophisticated biofeedback research on this topic. According to their studies, chronic alcoholics and children of alcoholics often have less alpha brainwave activity than non-alcoholic individuals. This finding suggests that a deficiency of alpha and theta brainwaves predisposes an individual to the development of alcoholism or other substance abuse.

Even more dramatic was their finding that alcohol enables many of these individuals to achieve alpha wave activity. This coincides with the suggestion by more and more authorities that addicts are searching for an experience of attunement, oneness, or inner harmony and peace, albeit in a dysfunctional manner. Furthermore, many unhealthy, compulsive behaviors such as alcohol abuse, smoking, overeating, caffeine consumption, and sexual addictions are actually the result of our inability to handle stress in our lives.

Thus the emerging field of addictionology seems to share a common denominator with the insights of philosophy, religion, and many spiritual traditions as well as of biophysics. Certain specific patterns of electrical brainwave activity are consistently in evidence when we feel a sense of "oneness" or deep peacefulness. This is true whether it is described in terms of profound relaxation or "mystical experience" or "connecting with one's Higher Power."

Other recent scientific discoveries suggest that there is a biological and electromagnetic reason why the brainwaves of deep relaxation and meditation are in the frequency range that they are. Geobiologist Joseph Kirschvink of the California Institute of Technology recently reported finding tiny magnets (actually, crystals of the mineral magnetite) in human brain tissue. The Earth itself has a specific harmonic resonance, pulsing at 8 cycles per second. When we become truly still, we allow our own electrical receiving apparatus (the neurons throughout our nervous system and brain) to align and attune to the Earth's own rhythm—an example of the law of rhythm entrainment. Perhaps this is the fundamental basis for the biblical adage, "Be still and know."

MUSIC TO THE RESCUE

If our bodies can resonate to the "music" of the Earth, whether we are listening or not, then it's not surprising that music we choose to hear can be one of the most effective paths to deep relaxation. Luckily for us, listening to music is a safe, time-tested, non-addictive, enjoyable way to relax—and one that doesn't require any special training. Bringing appropriate music and sounds into your life can help keep your physical and psychological being in tune. You can literally assist your cells and organs to relax and renew themselves, which will add more years to your life, as well as more life to your years.

Most music, from Bach to rock, is intended to stimulate rather than to relax. Its physiological effect is to dominate and override the natural rhythm of the heart by "entraining" it to the rhythm of the beat. Music that we seek out for relaxation was not necessarily written for that purpose, because we are only now learning what its action on our brainwaves is. There no reason not to take pleasure in both stimulating and relaxing music, but when the goal is "attunement" rather than "entertainment," only certain music possesses the characteristics needed to be effective.

In 1969, Steven Halpern, whom many consider to be the Father of New Age music, began developing an approach to composing that wasn't rock, pop, jazz, or classical. The music didn't have a dance beat and you couldn't hum the melody. But it had the ability to take the listener into a state of deep relaxation and inner peace.

In an interview, Steven told me, "I created a type of music that allows for a change in the energy fields of the body and also a change in brainwave patterns. My music is not about doing, it's about being. Listening to this music induces a person into a deeply relaxed state—an alpha brainwave state of 8 cycles per second, which is associated with feelings of serenity, joy, and well-being. When the body gets relaxed, there is an attunement to the natural pulsation of the body, which also happens to be 8 cycles per second. What happens electromagnetically in the body, around the head, is that you interact with the dominant electromagnetic fields of the planet. Literally, you link up into the larger power source of the planet."

Stringent scientific testing corroborates the positive relationship between listening to this type of music and accessing a relaxation state. Halpern cites a double-blind study in which his "Spectrum Suite" was played for one group of subjects and Liszt's "Liebestraum #3" for another. The listeners' brain waves and galvanic skin reaction were monitored, and their electromagnetic energy fields were recorded through Kirlian photography. Listeners to the Liszt piece showed minimal changes; listeners to "Spectrum Suite" showed radical changes in the direction of relaxation. A wide demographic selection of people were used in the study, but the response was uniform. Even people who didn't like Halpern's music demonstrated a relaxation response!

THE IMPACT OF MUSIC ON CELLS AND RELAXATION

A variety of scientists and lecturers at the Sixth International Montreux Congress on Stress, founded by Dr. Hans Selye and Dr. Norman Cousins, gave testimony to the connection between music and health. Music affects the electromagnetic field characteristics of the membrane of a cell. In fact, thanks to the discoveries of recent years, we know now that every cell in our bodies "moves" to the sounds of music. Traditional medicine is only just beginning to recognize how electromagnetic fields affect the entire body. A microscopic entity like a cell is so small that the amount of energy needed to affect it is minuscule.

Here is yet another way the physical world affects us at a most intimate level: it happens that, even though we may not consciously hear a noise, or we believe we can "tune out" that discordant, cacophonous music emanating from our neighbors' (or offspring's) speakers, our bodies do indeed respond. It's automatic. We resonate physically (e.g. increased blood pressure and emotional distress), as well as on the electromagnetic level.

Dr. Norman Shealy, a world-renowned former neurosurgeon and founding president of the American Holistic Medical Association, conducted a study in which his patients listened to specially chosen music, which included some classical selections as well as Halpern's "Spectrum Suite." The patients' levels of beta-endorphins rose dramatically. These endorphins are the natural mood enhancers that the body produces; they help us feel good and seem to produce a drug-free "natural high."

At Baltimore's St. Agnes Hospital, carefully selected classical music was provided in the intensive-care units. "Half an hour of music produced the same effect as ten milligrams of Valium," says Raymond Bahr, MD, head of the coronary-care unit. "Patients who had been awake for four straight days were able to go into a deep sleep." Other studies show that music can lower respiration rates, blood pressure, and basal metabolism, thus lessening physiological responses to stress. To increase your sense of serenity and balance, choose music that you enjoy and find calming. Then make sure you listen to that music at times of high stress during the day. In addition to using health-enhancing music to help you stay well in the face of everyday challenges to health and sanity, you will be taking responsibility for creating your own positive moods and feelings. You can then use this renewed and recharged energy state for any other work-related or personal pursuit. And with all the money you save by not getting sick and by operating at peak performance levels, you'll be able to expand your library of listening choices!

THE HEALING OR HARMFUL EFFECT OF MUSIC
Among the things I learned from Halpern about the health-giving powers of music is that on a physical, psychological, and energetic basis, some music can help promote the healing process, but other music is actually harmful. In order to appreciate how this works, it is necessary to understand four important points.

First, in order for there to be sound, something must vibrate. Whether we're talking about the human vocal cords or the strings of a piano, there is no sound without vibration. The principle of resonance relates to the way our bodies respond to the sound waves created by this vibration—the actual frequencies of particular tones, high or low. Different parts of our body resonate to different frequencies. Some of the therapeutic effects of sound and music are based on this principle of resonance.

Second, any continuous pulsation that we recognize as rhythm tends to cause our heartbeat and pulse to synchronize with it. This phenomenon is known as the principle of rhythm entrainment, which I've talked about. It is most significant, says Halpern, that some rhythms are in harmony with the natural pulsations of the body while others are not. Many of the more prevalent rhythms of today's music scene are not part of any organically based model and may produce negative effects, as Dr. John Diamond has demonstrated in his percipient book, *Your Body Doesn't Lie.*

Third, there are evidently psychological constructs that may be encoded into composition. These constructs tap psychological and emotional responses in listeners. The responses are by no means consistent, however. People's reactions to music are quite idiosyncratic, as we all know, and vary widely among listeners. Some people feel pleasure listening to heavy metal, and others feel pleasure listening to Beethoven. Halpern believes the pleasure principle and the endorphin response to music we enjoy come into play in this regard.

The fourth principle, which Halpern says overlays the others, is that of attunement. Are the sound stimuli to which they respond assisting listeners to move into more attunement—more complete harmony with themselves as physiological/emotional/ spiritual beings? Each of these principles, he believes, must be considered when we try to understand how sound and music promote or deter healing. Every style of music, be it old or new, African, Asian, or Western, has its own purpose and viability. Our job is to learn how to choose wisely what will increase our own health and happiness.

CHOOSE MUSIC WISELY

Traditional music therapy labels music as sedative or stimulative. These are broad enough categories, to be sure, but what is not generally known is that even these labels don't hold true for a significant percentage of the population. For instance, according to the Music Research Foundation's landmark studies, only about 55 percent of those who listened to a sedative and relaxing composition such as Liszt's "Leibestraum #3" found it to be sedative and relaxing. What about the other 45 percent? They found it stressful, perhaps, or stimulating. The problem is that there is no way to know beforehand, and this is one of the big problems with using existing classical music in therapeutic situations.

Another very important consideration in choosing music wisely was identified by Dr. John Diamond. After studying over 20,000 recordings, he found that different versions of the same composition might have radically different effects on listeners, due to the mood or energy imparted to that performance by that performer. Therefore, as Halpern points out, it is meaningless to say, "For relaxation, get some music by Mozart," as many writers do. At a minimum, one would need to designate which piece, and who performed it.

The whole issue is complicated by the fact that we may not be able to tell easily what our reaction is. For example, many people think they get relaxation from watching TV or listening to a Mozart symphony, but biofeedback measurements may prove that they are quite mistaken. In this case, belief does not equal fact.

There is one school of thought that suggests patients will receive the greatest relief from anxiety, insomnia, or whatever when allowed to listen to their favorite music, no matter what it is. Halpern has seen similar claims made for music selected to use during childbirth or during surgery. There's absurdity, even danger in this approach, according to Halpern. In choosing music for relaxation, which is a fundamental cornerstone of health and well-being, a person may easily ignore the well-established physiological parameters of relaxation. One of these is a relaxed heartbeat, which falls in the range of 60 beats per minute or less. Most music is faster than 60 beats per minute. So patients who think "Chariots of Fire," the theme music from *Rocky*, or selections from Bruce Springsteen will relax them are choosing out of habit and not from any knowledge of what is happening to their heartbeats.

In his book *Tuning the Human Instrument*, Halpern reported that more surgeons are starting to use specially composed relaxation music in surgery. Recently some surgeons stated that they like to operate with music, but only music of their choice. One of these surgeons likes country and western, another favors heavy metal. Remember rhythm entrainment? That means the blood of the patient would be pumping faster than normal—not what I would want if I were on the operating table. Clearly country and western and heavy metal are not designed for this context, because the physiological effects of the music conflict with the natural needs of the body.

The use of music during childbirth presents similar problems. The mother might like Springsteen's "Born in the USA," because the pounding rhythm gives her energy to push. But research reported at the International Pre- and Post-Perinatal Psychology Conference found that same rhythm can be terrible for the baby.

Not long ago, Halpern began composing music especially for children. He explains, "I was horrified to read that by the time a child is 18, he or she has already witnessed 20,000 TV murders. I believe we need influences that balance that stuff out. If parents provide a more harmonious, nurturing, soothing environment at home, even if they only play music at night when the children are sleeping, it helps." Parents have reported to him that their babies cry a lot less when his music is played.

One feature of music specially designed for relaxing is that it makes no demands on your attention. You may use it as background while you go about your work at home or at the office. Many people find this music especially helpful as a way to get centered at the start of the day and as a way of de-stressing after work, either during their commute or upon reaching home. In addition to enjoying any music by Josh Groban, the standards sung by Steve Tyrell or Rod Stewart, and a dozen other favorites, my best-loved "music" for de-stressing happens to be recorded sounds of nature, including gentle rain, ocean waves, babbling brooks, bird songs mixed with water sounds, breezes whispering in trees, etc. Some people play relaxing music during meals, while eating, reading, stretching, or working at a hobby, or while enjoying quiet moments with loved ones. Many find that it's easier to merge with the music when they use headphones to shut out other sounds. If you're using music specifically in order to relax, close your eyes, listen deeply, and let yourself become the music.

Visit your local music stores to see if they have recordings designed for relaxing, and check out specialty bookstores that may also carry New Age music and nature sounds. It's always best if the stores let you listen to anything available in the store before purchasing; some have headsets for that purpose.

It is now widely recognized that an innate drive in each of us seeks the experience of oneness, attunement, and inner harmony and peace. The better able we are to achieve that state on our own, the less we'll need to resort to alcohol, drugs, caffeine, or other forms of addictive behavior as distorted expressions of the search for serenity. True healing involves integration and attunement with oneself and one's world. What has been forgotten in much of the criticism of New Age music is that its most serious practitioners focus on the goal of using sound and music as a vehicle for bringing us into a state of inner peace and harmony. Using music as the gateway to silence and stillness may seem like a paradox, but what might be considered the "other-worldly" quality of both New Age music and "old" Gregorian chant suggests that it truly is a gateway. By turning inward, we are reminded who and what we really are.

When we become still, as we do in a state of deep relaxation, meditation, or prayer, we allow our own electromagnetic receiving apparatus—our body, mind, and spirit—to align and attune to the fundamental frequency of the Earth itself, because this frequency is in the precise range of our deep alpha brainwave activity. The electromagnetic field created by our own electrical nervous system entrains to the electromagnetic field of the Earth. What can be more natural than that? It's like allowing the human instrument to tune and play itself more effectively. Music that assists in attaining alpha or theta frequencies can help each of us, on an individual basis, experience a greater sense of wholeness, oneness, and attunement.

In addition, when two or more of us are tuned into this gentle vibration of Love and Light, we help amplify others' entrainment to this state. Individual entrainment thus enhances collective entrainment. In other words, as we experience inner peace and harmony within ourselves, we actually establish and emanate a harmonic vibration with which others can resonate. This may ultimately be the greatest gift music has to offer. It can help each of us take responsibility for ourselves and do what we can to create more relaxing, peaceful, happy lives.

The bottom line is this: No matter what your musical taste, therapeutic music is any music that enhances the built-in healing modalities of the body. We are fooling ourselves and wasting our time, says Halpern, with anything else. The problem is that very few truly relaxing and healing albums ever make it onto the charts. If you enjoy the music of Enya, for instance, which is often considered relaxing even though it's popular, it's not what you'd listen to when you desire total relaxation. If you are skilled in recognizing the feedback from your body/mind, and are experienced in identifying therapeutic and positive effects, and if you've done your homework, you can trust your instincts. If not, trust the professionals—the artists and therapists who devote their lives to the work of producing music with therapeutic effects.

RELAXATION: A KEY TO HEALING AND ATTUNEMENT

As I mentioned earlier, recent discoveries in brain science suggest that all of us require at least 30 minutes each day during which the brain's electrical activity registers in the alpha (8–12 cps) and theta (4–7 cps) ranges. Listening to appropriate music is one of the easiest, most effective and enjoyable ways to ensure that you're getting your Minimum Daily Requirement. But, once again, not just any music will do.

The amazing popularity of Gregorian chant, to which I listen often, suggests that it may fill the basic requirement for brain health and happiness. This music didn't come about by chance; it was composed in a sacred context, and the elements of positive intent and dedicated performance have resulted in centuries of proven healing and uplifting effect. New Age music that is inspired by therapeutic, beneficial motives can be understood as a contemporary expression of the ancient tradition that gave us Gregorian chant.

Am I recommending that you stop listening to music that doesn't elicit a relaxation response? Absolutely not! I enjoy listening to all kinds of music, including rock, jazz, easy listening, country, show tunes, and classical. In fact, there's a different benefit to these more complex types of music, according to psychologist Frances Rauscher, PhD, and neuroscientist Gordon Shaw, PhD, of the University of California at Irvine. They say that complex music enhances our spatial intelligence—the ability to "see" the world accurately. They have shown that the spatial IQ scores of college students go up after hearing ten minutes of a Mozart sonata and that musically inclined preschoolers' puzzle-building skills improve as well.

Dancing and singing, two of the greatest activities in the world, are also as therapeutic as they are enjoyable. When you're dancing or singing, you are feeling rhythm entrainment and resonance at a conscious level, releasing stress, and increasing the body's beta-endorphins, even though you may think you're just having fun. Ellen DeGeneres would probably agree. Her love of dancing and singing, combined with her ebullient attitude on her TV talk show, brings such joy and happiness to all the viewers and makes everyone watching feel like dancing (at least I do!). Pick any piece of music that makes you want to move, and go with it. Sing along with your favorite rock, pop, or opera star. I was once told by a wise mentor and teacher, "It's impossible to sing and feel sorry for yourself at the same time!" If you think you're not at performance level and would prefer not to be seen or heard, go into a room by yourself and close the door before you turn on the radio.

Listening to music, any music, is another way you can learn to be in tune with your body's reactions. Whether you're responding in a packed concert venue or in the solitary haven of headphones, you're experiencing rhythm, harmony, and the amazing potency of sounds. Music also trains the ears to hear musical, healing sounds in the natural world. In fact, composers for centuries have paid tribute to nature's sounds—wind, ocean waves, bird songs, whale and dolphin communications—and have taken advantage of their particular magic. So enjoy whatever music you wish; just be sure to choose carefully when it comes to relaxation and attunement.

Each patient carries his own doctor inside him.
—ALBERT SCHWEITZER

Do not go where the path may lead. Go instead where there is no path and leave a trail.
—RALPH WALDO EMERSON

Chapter 5

Exercise—Fast and Slow, Alone and Together
I Choose to Move!

I wish that life should not be cheap, but sacred.
I wish the days to be as centuries, loaded, fragrant.
—Ralph Waldo Emerson
I still get wildly enthusiastic about little things . . .
I paly with leaves, I skip down the street and against the
wind.
—Leo Buscaglia

We all know exercise is a key component of vibrant health, yet statistics reveal that only about 25 percent of Americans make exercise a regular part of their lifestyle. My hope is that after reading this chapter, if you're not already a fitness enthusiast, you'll be helping to increase the percentage. Whether you have several children and are busy with them from morning to night or are CEO of a Fortune 500 company who puts in 10 to 12 hours a day, seven days a week at the job, you must find time to exercise.

If you can't carve out an hour each day to exercise, or even 30 minutes, then break the time up into 10- or 15-minute allotments. It should be pretty clear by now that I don't believe in gimmicks and potions and magic pills, and I promise you there is no substitute for exercise. The old "I don't have time to exercise" excuse just doesn't work with me. You must make fitness a priority—a nonnegotiable part of your day.

You need—we all need—to find some type of physical activity that fits into your lifestyle and that exercises not only your body but also your mind and spirit. If there is one self-help idea that has really caught on and that I'm sure will stay with us, it's the idea that physical fitness transcends the physical body and benefits your mental and spiritual fitness as well.

STAYING MOTIVATED TO EXERCISE

Kim used to do all her workouts in the gym. Four to five mornings a week, before dawn, she went to her gym and walked on the treadmill, staring out into space, oblivious to her immediate environment. I saw her doing the same 45 minutes on the treadmill for weeks, only occasionally switching to the bike or the stair climber. Then one day, after her workout was complete, I introduced myself and told her I had just finished my strength training routine. I asked her about her workout. She admitted to me that although what she did was convenient and gave her good results, it was boring. "I am a morning person, so it's not too hard getting up before the rest of the world," she said to me, "but it's often hard to motivate myself to get on the treadmill and do the same old thing."

Then she asked what I liked to do for my cardio training, so I told her about my passion for hiking and being outdoors. "There's something about being in nature, feeling the sun, breathing the fresh air, absorbing the mood-lifting negative ions, and actually going somewhere, as opposed to walking in place, that makes the time fly and makes the workout fun," I told Kim. She was intrigued, and I asked her if she would like to accompany me on a hike the following morning.

We agreed to meet at the head of one of the Santa Monica trails, just minutes from both of our homes, at 6 a.m., the same time as her usual workout. Her experience was no different from that of my many other friends who started in the gym and are now avid hikers. While hiking you can take in a variety of terrain, flora, and fauna and soak up a wide range of sensations, sights, sounds, and scents as you move and work out your entire body. Hiking strengthens your body and feeds your soul. Of course, seasonal and weather changes offer further variety as your program continues throughout the year, as does an occasional change of location. For three decades I've told my clients and friends that making exercise fun should be as high a priority as making it effective. And even if you don't live in a climate that's conducive to exercising outdoors year-round, you can still add fun into workouts simply by listening to terrific music, going to a gym that motivates you, watching an exercise DVD that's invigorating, parking at the end of a parking lot, and walking faster to your location. I do this frequently when I travel and still want to get in some exercise. Lightweight and easily packed exercise bands and an upbeat music CD can do wonders for hotel room workouts.

MAKE IT SOCIAL

Another reason I love to hike is that it's easier to make exercise a social experience in the outdoors. Often my days are filled with activities and responsibilities, and when I do have time to visit with my friends, it's usually over a meal at a restaurant. When I hike with a friend, however, we get to spend real quality time together as we super-tune our bodies, minds, and spirits. And we get to burn calories instead of adding calories as we would if we were getting together over lunch or dinner.

My favorite time to hike is in the early morning. The time passes more quickly outdoors, which makes it easier to do a longer workout. I get so absorbed in what I'm doing, seeing, hearing, feeling, and saying that when I'm done, I feel completely relaxed and energized at the same time, and I'm ready to take on the world.

You can make your workout more intense by finding some hills, increasing your pace, or inviting a very fit hiking partner who will push you harder. As a personal fitness trainer for over 30 years, I've seen what happens when clients or friends elect to work out solely in the gym. They often experience burnout. The attrition rate tends to be high for exercise programs in the gym, whether people are simply lifting weights or are taking different kinds of classes. The chances of quitting are much lower for those who exercise outdoors at least once or twice a week. If you don't live in close proximity to any hiking trails, there are other activities you can do outdoors to help achieve a balance of physical, mental, and spiritual fitness: walking, running or jogging, in-line skating, kayaking, cross-country skiing, road cycling, mountain biking, swimming, and skiing are some examples. The activity you choose depends on preference and convenience. If you've enjoyed doing one particular form of outdoor exercise in the past, your choice might be simple, but you might also enjoy trying something different. I exhort you to move out of your comfort zone when it comes to your workouts, and try something new. Often you are more inspired to embark on a new activity when you're with a friend.

A few friends of mine are too busy during the week to hike, swim, or mountain bike, so they leave these activities for the weekend. Weekend outdoor workouts afford you the greatest time flexibility, but if you happen to work near a park or some other appropriate venue, an invigorating lunch-hour run or skate could be the perfect cardio solution for you. If you happen to live in a pedestrian-friendly neighborhood, try taking a brisk walk from your home. Map out a route, with some hills if possible, so that you know how long it takes and can schedule it in during the day. For my workout, I love going to the most expensive neighborhoods and inspecting the variety of resplendent gardens and architectural styles as I go by. When I'm appreciating the passing scene (and sometimes rearranging or upgrading the gardens in my mind), time seems to go quickly. Before I know it I've walked an hour or more, and I feel renewed and empowered because I kept my word to work out and at the same time enjoyed some uplifting scenery.

The principles of a good workout program are exactly the same outdoors as they are in the health club. Start slowly, build gradually, and keep challenging yourself. If you're a beginner, learn proper technique from a class or an experienced friend in order to exercise better and avoid injury. If you've never been hiking before, make sure you go with someone who can show you the trails, guide you in your technique, and help you appreciate the exquisiteness of your environment. Always seek help with a sport you haven't tried before.

As I have written in detail in my book, *Health Bliss*, whatever activity you choose outdoors, remember to warm up and cool down with five minutes of low-intensity activity and to work out at least 20 minutes at your fat-burning target heart rate. You might want to look into getting a heart rate monitor to use outdoors if you can't easily calculate your exercising heart rate. Remember, too, that if one of your goals is to lose fat, you need to work up to at least 45 minutes of cardio each session, because the body burns more fat as fuel when you work out for longer than 20 minutes. Beginners, please increase gradually until you reach the extended time.

Make sure you dress appropriately when you exercise outdoors. Always wear clothing that has been designed for the activity you're doing and is suitable for any weather conditions you might encounter. Always use sunscreen when needed, and hydrate your body with plenty of pure water before and after your workout—during it if you work out longer than one hour.

MARATHON MYSTERY

I ran my first marathon in the Los Angeles area, after devoting a whole year to training, during the first week of December 1975. When race day arrived, my emotions were mixed. On the one hand, I was excited and eager to run, although I wasn't quite sure what to expect since I had never embarked on an endurance event before. On the other hand, I was feeling melancholy because that day was the one-year anniversary of my grandmother Fritzie's death. Fritzie had taught me much of what I knew about spirituality, self-reliance, simplicity, and living fully. As I was driving to Culver City the morning of the race, I felt a tremendous longing to visit with her. I missed her so much that I was actually talking out loud to her in the car as a way to soothe the ache in my heart. I even said that I was open to her spirit and energy and asked her to let me know somehow, some way, if she could hear me. I also asked her to help me run the marathon and complete it.

When I arrived at the starting location, there were lots of people getting ready. I wished there was just one person I knew, so I wouldn't have to run alone. The starting gun went off, and so did a few thousand runners. For the first three miles I ran alone and felt great—confident, relaxed, and energetic. Sometime during the fourth mile, a young man who looked to be in his mid-twenties ran up next to me and we began talking. Before we knew it, we were at mile 10, then 15, then 20. It's amazing the things you'll tell someone you've never met before when you are running together. It must have something to do with the release of certain chemicals in the body and a change in the electrical activity of the brain during aerobic exercise. We talked about our lives, families,

The Joy Factor

interests, dreams, and goals. I was feeling extremely grateful to him because our conversation made the miles sail by.

Before we knew it, we were at mile 25. At this point we started talking about where we lived, and when he told me he lived in Studio City I said, "That's interesting. My grandmother used to live in Studio City. What street do you live on?" The name of the street made me gasp. It was the same street Fritzie had lived on. We were close to the finish, and I had barely enough time to inquire about his exact location before we crossed the finish line. He told me just as we crossed that he had moved into an apartment there eleven months earlier, and that the lady who lived there before him had passed away. I could hardly breathe—not because I was tired, but because of what he was telling me: he had moved into Fritzie's apartment.

Out of all the thousands of people in the race, I ended up running and sharing mutual support with the person who now lived in my grandmother's apartment—and it was only a few hours after I had asked Fritzie for some sign that she was receiving my communication. Coincidence? I think not. The physical and the spiritual mingle all the time if we believe, have faith, and trust our inner guidance.

SLOW DOWN WITH YOGA

In this age of moving fast, eating fast, and doing everything at breakneck speed, people need ways of slowing down enough to hear that inner guidance. Yoga, an ancient mind/body discipline from India, is one of the best slowing-down mechanisms I know. It is both strenuous and peaceful; an old way of seeking the quiet place inside ourselves that seems startlingly new. It has become so popular, I believe, because it combines physical exercise with a mental and spiritual focus. Yoga is the opposite of aerobic exercise in that it slows the pace of life, if only for an hour. In that hour we pay attention to the totality of who we are and concentrate on stretching and strengthening the body, mind, and spirit.

When I first started to practice yoga, I began working with videotapes or DVDs at home so that I could feel a little more comfortable attending a class. I liked the idea of trying some poses first in the privacy of my home, but I soon discovered that I appreciated the supportive environment of a good yoga studio and instructor. If you've never tried yoga before, I encourage you to do so. It's helpful to learn with a real live teacher, but you can do a lot on your own.

Think for a minute about our day-to-day range of motion. It is usually limited to familiar positions and familiar movements— sitting, standing, lying down, walking, or bending a little. We are capable of so much more. Practicing the different yoga poses, or asanas, takes the body into every position it can possibly assume. By doing that, it opens up different perspectives, both of moving and of thinking. These motions release the tensions in the body, sending clarifying signals through our neurological pathways and promoting creativity.

In yoga, through a combination of poses, deep breathing, body awareness, and focus, you learn that your life is right here, right now. In other words, you come to appreciate the power of the present moment. You can't be thinking about paying bills or picking children up from school if you have to stand steady in a balancing posture or stretch correctly in a forward bend. If your mind is elsewhere, you cannot perform the movement well. Yoga teaches you to live fully in the present, instead of digressing into the past or future or into the imagination. Yoga has helped me to pour my energy fully into the moment. It's all about being fully alive and fully present.

About ten years ago I was flying from Los Angeles to Monterey to give a motivational talk. During the flight I sat next to a man and we started talking about our lives and our favorite activities for fitness and relaxation. When I told him that I enjoyed yoga, his attitude toward me changed instantly from positive to negative, just as if I'd flipped a switch. Surprised, I asked him what was wrong. He told me that yoga was a phony, outlandish religion and he would never have anything to do with it. Then he got up and moved to the back of the plane. I must admit I was baffled. Never before had I encountered that particular response, and it was apparent that the man was completely ignorant about yoga. Had he stayed in his seat beside me, I would have told him that yoga is not a religion. Yoga, which means "union with God," is a tool for delving deeper into whatever your own true beliefs and interests are. Whether you are of the Jewish, Catholic, Protestant, Buddhist, Muslim or any other faith, yoga helps you express your own philosophy with balance and serenity—in your body and in your life. By increasing the flexibility of your body, you can thwart the hardening of your attitudes and by eschewing patterned, judgmental thinking, you can strengthen and tone your mind and heart.

There is no better remedy for stress than yoga, and no better non-cardiac exercise. If you aren't already practicing this challenging but enjoyable discipline, make it a point to attend a beginning class or check out a video from your library. It will enrich and nurture all aspects of your body and life.

PRAYER-WALKING AND HIKING

If you're looking for a more aerobic activity that goes beyond mere physical exercise to improve the fitness of mind, body, and spirit, prayer-walking is for you. Monks have been doing it for centuries, but now it's catching on in the mainstream. I've been doing prayer-walks and hikes for three decades, but only recently have I come across a book that beautifully expresses this practice that has truly blessed my life. The book is *Prayer-Walking—A Simple Path to Body-and-Soul Fitness* by Linus Mundy. He describes prayer-walking as taking a stroll with your soul: a simple, natural prescription for growing spiritually while you're "going" physically. Jesus and Gandhi both did it, and for our hectic, "busyness" lifestyles it's the perfect antidote. I find it a winning combination that improves my health and well-being and nourishes my mind and soul at the same time. For those of you who are into multitasking and making good use of your oh-so-limited time, this concept of combining walking and prayer should be most appealing.

Prayer-walking eliminates the artificial separation of the spiritual and physical realms. You don't have to kneel or even go to church in order to pray. You can pray while making dinner, driving a car, eating lunch, digging in the garden, changing diapers, or enjoying a quiet moment. What matters is communicating with God and experiencing God in and all around you. Most of us are busy talking all day long. Just 20 minutes of walking in silent contemplation can slow down the mind, relax the body, and feed the soul. Besides, it's a practical and efficient way to preclude overloading the daily schedule!

"Deciding to take a prayer-walk means scheduling a time and a place where God can touch us and we can touch God," writes Mundy. There is no right way and no wrong way to prayer-walk. He recommends a five-step approach to finding body-soul fitness. The first step is to retreat—go someplace to walk, preferably in a natural setting. If that's not possible, the mall or the sidewalk will do. "Prayer-walking can teach us that it's all holy ground we walk on, whether that ground is in the laundry room, in the boardroom, or under roomy skies."

The second step is to rethink—give our minds a break from everyday burdens and focus on the present through prayer. The third is to remember and reinvent community walks or processions. The memory of any such experiences you may have had can be inspiring. If you have never done this, you might join with any local group that is walking for a reason or to a place with special meaning for you.

The fourth step is to repent. Mundy is quick to point out that this word is fraught with connotations. He uses it in the sense of engaging in self-examination and assessing our own behavior to see where we might improve ourselves. "Who doesn't want to become a better person?" he asks. The last step, and perhaps the most important, is to repeat. To reap the rewards of prayer-walking, Mundy says, "I cannot overemphasize the importance of setting a schedule and sticking to it."

When I teach this kind of walking, I tell beginners to start with 20 minutes at least three times a week. Make sure to walk fast enough to elevate your heart rate so that you will get a workout. (Please refer to my books, *Recipes for Health Bliss: Using NatureFoods & Lifestyle Choices to Rejuvenate Your Body & Life* and *Health Bliss: 50 Revitalizing NatureFoods & Lifestyle Choices to Promote Vibrant Health,* for more information in exercise, accelerating fat loss, ramping up metabolism, and the power foods you'll want to eat to create a fit, lean body.) Of course, if you're not a beginner you can walk longer for more benefits. On days when, for whatever reason, you don't feel like walking fast, it's all right to go at a more leisurely pace.

During your walk, pick one of your favorite affirmations, or mantras, or prayers. It should be short, easy to say, and meaningful for you. This mantra is something each individual should choose. For some it might be "Thy will be done," or "This day I live in perfect peace." For others "Shalom" or "Hail Mary" might work best. Mundy suggests that you pick a phrase that pertains to your own tradition or one that suits your own tastes and interests. Atheists and agnostics can participate with mantras such as "Live Fully," "Peace-Joy," or "Still-Ness." There are so many possibilities; you could choose a different one for every day of the year.

"It is not what is said that matters," says Herbert Benson, MD, director of the Mind/Body Medicine Institute of the Harvard Medical School. "It is the repetition of a key phrase which triggers the health benefits." He did point out that what is said matters a great deal to the person saying it, and that a phrase with which the individual was not comfortable would create tension and undermine the benefits.

And the benefits are impressive indeed. Several years ago Benson and James Rippe, MD, then of the University of Massachusetts at Worcester, conducted a study in which the participants did a standard fitness walking program and focused their minds at the same time. "We found it was possible for them to elicit the relaxation response while exercising, and thus get the benefits of both at once." In the 1960s and 70s, as Benson wrote in his ground-breaking book, *The Relaxation Response*, the researchers saw indisputable evidence that meditation and prayer elevate one's mood and produce beneficial physiological effects, including a slower heart rate, lower blood pressure, and key hormonal changes.

"Our subjects [in the focused walking study] concentrated on their footfall, but the principle is the same as if they had been praying. Their focus brought on the relaxation response. They felt better after the walk than they would have just walking alone. They derived the same degree of cardiovascular training but had a measurable boost in mood and a reduction in stress. One of the few drawbacks to exercise is that it can produce a stress effect. The relaxation response neutralizes that." In his studies, Benson has observed a 36 percent reduction in people's doctor bills that could be attributed to prayer and meditation. He is convinced prayer-walking might lead to a significant reduction in spiraling medical costs—for individuals and society.

When I do prayer-walking, I select places in nature, whether in the mountains, by the ocean, in the desert, or at a botanical garden or local park. I try to find areas with the least noise and the fewest people, especially places where I won't run into anyone I know. It can be very disconcerting, when you've been prayer-walking for 20 or 30 minutes and are deeply into your inner reflection, to hear someone call your name and come over for a chat. If that happens, politely say that you're doing a special silent workout today and will be happy to give them a call later on. That usually works. If not, enjoy the encounter and then pick up where you left off, or try again another day.

What I've learned about prayer-walking is even more true of prayer-hiking. Prayer-hiking is the ultimate experience for me, because I'm enveloped in the musical sounds of nature, the majesty of the trees, the fresh air, the fragrance of the surroundings, and the subtle whisperings of the angelic forces all around. When I make my hike a prayer-hike, I choose paths I know well so that my mind won't deviate from its inner focus to figure out which way to go. Since I've hiked the Santa Monica Mountains for three decades, I know the idiosyncracies and nuances of all the different trails very well. You can conduct a prayer-hike with a friend or two, knowing that you'll choose silence during the hike and catch up on things when the hike is over. If you can't resist conversation when a friend is around, however, you might choose to prayer-hike alone in order to garner the most benefits for body, mind, and spirit.

By silently communing with what is around us, we can learn many things, and this is especially true when it comes to prayer-hiking. Sometimes, instead of repeating an affirmation or mantra, I will simply stay in the present during the hike, breathe deeply, and focus on and appreciate the beauty all around me. This is much harder to do than you might think. When I first started doing it, my mind seemed to wander every few seconds like an untrained puppy, to every subject but the task at hand— appreciating the beauty of my surroundings. It took about a year, prayer-hiking four to six times monthly, for me to be able to do an entire one- or two-hour hike absorbed in nothing but the present and the beauty around me. Like anything worth learning, prayer-hiking takes disciplined practice, but the effort has made a positive, profound difference in all areas of my life. The physical and mental discipline brings spiritual discipline, and when all three are in harmony, all directed by the same desire and intention, I feel faith-filled, empowered, and invincible. And, most important to me, I feel divinely guided and loved by God and my angels and guides and connected to everything good and loving.

Turn on any news program or read any newspaper and you'll doubtless find information abounding on crime, terrorism, violence, war, and every kind of abuse. The information alone is enough to create within us fear, frustration, confusion, and disharmony. The most effective way I know to restore balance and foster serenity is to appreciate beauty. Of course you can visit a museum, listen to a symphony, watch an awe-inspiring movie, or arrange some freshly cut flowers in your home, but I think simply being out in nature is the best. The natural environment is the most fundamental form of beauty, and it's absolutely free. When you are "out of sorts" and need to be reconnected with your own true beauty and best self, nature will gently steer you in the right direction. Our hearts and minds resonate with the amazing colors and sounds of nature, and our cells actually begin to vibrate at a higher frequency that affords a deeper spiritual connection and a feeling of belonging.

Nature is also rich in the vitamins of the air. The air we breathe contains a large number of good and bad compounds, some of which are essential nutrients in the form of vitamins, minerals, and trace elements. Air is much like food—there is "junk" air and "healthy" air to breathe. Bad air vitiates the functioning of mind and body, while good air, like good food, awakens the senses and enlivens the being. Noxious or junk air is full of positive ions, but healthy air is charged with many negative ions. (Ions are atoms or molecules with a net electric charge due to the loss or gain of one or more electrons.) Indoor environments such as our offices, cars, and homes are all but devoid of valuable breathable nutrients, including negative ions, which are needed for the proper absorption of oxygen (and have repeatedly been shown to help combat depression, improve respiratory problems, prevent migraines and other headaches, combat fatigue, etc.). Nature provides an abundance of negative ions near waterfalls, by the ocean, in the mountains, around trees and other plants, and after a good thunderstorm. Increasing the negative ions you inhale can help you feel better, look younger, and live longer. Spend as much time out in nature as you possibly can and bring nature (and negative ions) into your home with living plants and fountains.

Yes, we can learn so much from Mother Nature. She shows us the rhythm of the seasons and the balance of existence. She shows us the importance of times of withdrawal in attaining peace and serenity; the necessity of acceptance—flowing with the conditions of life; the wise use of energy and play; the true freedom that comes from lack of self-consciousness; and the strength that comes from being totally in the present.

Another reason I love to go hiking and conduct my prayer-hikes is the joy I feel being where there are trees—lots of trees. They are magical for me. Trees provide us with beauty, shade, oxygen, and wisdom. Yes, wisdom. Find a beautiful tree that calls out to you the next time you're hiking or are in a garden. Maybe it's an old tree in your yard. Wherever it is, walk over to it, wrap your arms around it, and give it a big hug and kiss. I'm pretty sure you'll laugh, or at least smile. Then put your back to the tree and for five minutes breathe deeply, eyes closed, thanking the tree for its presence and beauty. Next, if you have any questions that need to be answered about things going on in your life, silently ask the tree for its guidance. I've been doing this for years, especially when hiking, and have invariably received answers that gave me the courage and strength to make necessary changes in my life. Be patient. Maybe you won't hear and feel a response right away. Sometimes it's been a day or two before the answers came to me.

White Eagle writes about trees in his inspiring book, *Walking with the Angels*:

The trees enfold humanity as a mother;
the trees are symbolic of the great Mother.
Realize this, we can walk in the groves, sit beneath the great oaks,
or an ancient banyan, or the majesty of the cedar, and become conscious
of this divine mother-love enfolding us.
The sages of old chose the trees as their cathedrals.
Can you not recognize in the pillar and arch and groyne of
the cathedral or palace, a symbol or a replica of the fundamental principles of the structure of a tree? In some quiet woodland—
veritably a natural cathedral—have you not felt the sense of love and

peace, and registered the blessing of those natural sanctuaries?
There are many such cathedrals built by the tree spirits
on the astral plane of life,
where many weary souls coming from the earth can find refreshment
and worship, not by word, but through the adoration
and thankfulness of their hearts.

White Eagle beautifully describes how I feel when I hike. I feel so loved and blessed, so grateful and appreciative of life, so deeply connected to my spirituality and my Higher Self. I feel divinely protected and guided. I also feel mighty and powerful, knowing that whatever the world brings to me that day, I can handle it because I'm never alone. I don't get those feelings when I work out in a health club. The gym has its place, or course, and I go to mine two to four times a week for weight training when I'm not traveling. But I always make sure I carve out time to do workouts in nature, because this type of workout feeds my soul.

Spending time in nature can do this for you, too. Whether you choose to prayer-walk or hike, or simply find a place outdoors in nature to work out, you will strengthen your body, mind, and spirit and this whole-person integration will enrich every area of your life. In other words, nothing will do more good for you in terms of being vibrantly healthy, energetic, and youthful than a consistent, well-rounded fitness program that nourishes your body and soul.

Your work is to discover your work and then with all your heart to give yourself to it.
—BUDDHA

Anxiety is the mark of spiritual insecurity.
—THOMAS MERTON

CHAPTER 6

Deepen Your Relationship with Yourself

I CHOOSE TIME FOR REFLECTION

I love those who yearn for the impossible.
—JOHANN WOLFGANG VON GOETHE

To see the world in a grain of sand,
And heaven in a wild flower,
Hold infinity in the palm of your hand,
And eternity in an hour.
—WILLIAM BLAKE

Another practice that brings out our vitality and keeps us tuned into ourselves and connected with our source is meditation. Meditation is an ancient art that goes back long before recorded history. Stone seals dating back to at least 5,000 BC have been found in the Indus Valley of India, showing people seated in various yoga postures. For all these millennia, meditation has survived as a vital science of living. This is not because meditation is esoteric or exotic or exclusively for monks and yogis, but because anybody can do it, and the benefits are perfectly clear to anybody who observes them.

Only during the past three decades, however, has scientific study focused on the clinical effects of meditation on health. The August 4, 2003 cover story of *Time* by Joel Stein was titled "The Science of Meditation" with the caption: "New Age mumbo jumbo? Not for millions of Americans who meditate for health and well-being." Scientists study it; doctors recommend it; millions of Americans—many of whom don't even own crystals—practice it daily. Why? Because meditation works! In fact, scientists have now developed tools sophisticated enough to see what goes on in your brain when you engage in a consistent meditation program.

In a nutshell: One study found that after training in meditation for eight weeks, subjects showed a pronounced change in brain-wave patterns, shifting from the beta waves of aroused, conscious thought to the alpha and theta waves that dominate the brain during periods of deep relaxation. Sound intriguing? Read on.

Meditation is so thoroughly effective in reducing stress and tension, for example, that in 1984 the National Institutes of Health recommended meditation over prescription drugs as the first treatment for mild hypertension. The late Dr. Hans Selye, a pioneering Canadian stress researcher, described two types of stress: negative stress and positive stress. The difference between the two depends upon whether or not we feel in control of the stress. Meditation, by making us more aware of our reactions to stress, can lead us toward an increased internal sense of control.

HEALTH BENEFITS OF MEDITATION

Dr. R. Keith Wallace at the University of California, Los Angeles, conducted the first research on the physiology of meditation. Studying Transcendental Meditation, Wallace found that during meditation the body arrives at a state of profound rest while the brain and mind become more alert, indicating a state of "restful alertness." Studies showed that after meditation, people exhibit faster reactions, greater creativity, and broader comprehension. Dr. Herbert Benson of the Mind-Body Institute at Harvard University determined that meditation practice can bring about a healthy state of relaxation by causing a generalized reduction in physiological and biochemical stress indicators. Among the favorable indications are decreased heart rate, decreased respiration rate, decreased plasma cortisol (a stress hormone), decreased pulse rate, increased alpha waves (a brain wave associated with relaxation), and increased oxygen consumption.

Scientists are finding that meditation also helps keep us young and wrinkle-free. One study showed that people who had been meditating for more than five years were biologically 12 to 15 years younger than people who don't meditate. A comparison of the hospital records of 2,000 meditators and 2,000 non-meditators revealed that the meditators required only half as much medical care. They had 87 percent less heart disease, 55 percent fewer tumors, and 87 percent fewer nervous disorders. Just a few of the benefits of meditation are:

- Faster reaction time
- Greater creativity
- Broader comprehension
- Lowered stress
- Decreased heart rate
- Decreased respiration rate
- Decreased cortisol
- Decreased pulse rate
- Increase in alpha waves in the brain (key to relaxation)
- Increased oxygen consumption

Another medical expert who advocates meditation is Dean Ornish, MD, a well-known physician and author of many books. In his path-paving book, *Dr. Dean Ornish's Program for Reversing Heart Disease*, there are easy-to-follow instructions for a calming routine that includes meditation, yoga, and progressive relaxation. So effective is his program that I sent my mother to attend one of his seven-day residential lifestyle retreats in Northern California; she returned with a new glow and commitment to healthy living.

Jon Kabat-Zinn, MD, at the University of Massachusetts Medical School, author of *Wherever You Go There You Are*, founded the Stress Reduction Clinic in 1979 to help people suffering from chronic pain and chronic diseases such as cancer and heart disease, as well as stress-related disorders such as abdominal pain, chronic diarrhea, and ulcers. According to Dr. Kabat-Zinn, these conditions are often the most difficult to treat, and the patients have frequently tried other, more conventional forms of medicine without complete success.

Kabat-Zinn designed a stress-reduction program to test the value of using mindfulness meditation as an aid to patients in developing effective coping strategies for stress, and to see whether meditation would have any effect on their various chronic medical conditions. His stress-reduction program patients had to make a commitment to practice on their own each day. As it turned out, the majority of people improved in a number of different ways.

- Virtually all patients, whatever their diagnoses, showed a dramatic reduction in physical symptoms over the eight-week period.
- Psychological problems—anxiety, depression, hostility— also dropped over the eight weeks. Follow-up studies four years after completion of the course showed that both physical and psychological improvements were consistent over time.
- Symptom reductions were greater than with other techniques such as drug intervention, indicating that the results were not coming from a placebo effect. Somehow the patients' inner resources for healing were being tapped.
- Patients' self-perceptions changed. They viewed themselves as healthier and better able to handle stressful situations without suffering destructive effects. They felt more in control of their lives, viewed life as a challenge rather than as a series of obstacles, and felt they were living more fully.

In general, Kabat-Zinn concludes that meditation is effective in decreasing pain, reducing the secretion of stress hormones including adrenaline and noradrenaline, decreasing the amount of excess stomach acid in people with gastrointestinal problems, lowering blood pressure, and increasing relaxation.

MANAGING CANCER WITH MEDITATION

A new study from the Tom Baker Cancer Centre in Calgary has shown that meditation can substantially reduce levels of emotional distress and stress-related symptoms like headache, muscle tension, and stomach upset in patients undergoing chemotherapy.

As reported in *Psychosomatic Medicine*, researchers randomly assigned 90 cancer patients to one of two groups. The first group attended a meditation class once a week for seven weeks and was encouraged to meditate at least 30 minutes daily at home. The second group did not attend classes or receive instruction. Those who meditated experienced a major reduction in feelings of anger, depression, fatigue, and anxiety, and enjoyed a 31 percent drop in headaches, digestive problems, and racing heart.

MEDITATION AND THE BREATH

Although there are many approaches to meditation, they can generally be grouped into two basic techniques: concentrative meditation and mindfulness meditation. Both are directed toward focusing the attention and strengthening the concentration, with the goal of quieting the mind to stillness.

Concentrative meditation focuses the attention on the breath, on an image, or on a sound (mantra) in order to slow the mind's activity and allow a greater awareness and clarity to emerge. To sit quietly and focus on your breath is the simplest form of concentrative meditation. This technique of meditation can be compared to the zoom lens of a camera that narrows its focus to a selected field.

Concentration is the ability to tell yourself to pay attention to something and then do exactly that! Our errant minds tend to drift. We have continuous mental conversations. Most people talk to themselves nearly every minute of the day. Through meditation we can limit, control, and finally eliminate this internal chitchat.

An effective way to control and master your mind is through breath awareness. The connection between the breath and one's state of mind is a basic principle of both yoga and meditation. Think back to a time when you were frightened, agitated, distracted, or anxious. Whether or not you noticed it then, your breath was probably shallow, rapid, and uneven, and you could probably duplicate those stressful emotions simply by breathing in a ragged, arrhythmic way. When the mind is focused and composed, the breath tends to be slow, deep, and regular. Working in reverse in just the same way, you can calm your mind by consciously taking slow, deep, and regular breaths. The continuous rhythm of inhalation and exhalation provides a natural focus for the mind, which facilitates meditation.

Breath control is an amazing tool that allows you to alter your existing mental state. Inhale slowly and rhythmically through your nose, breathing quietly and deliberately. The incoming breath fills, in sequence, the abdomen, the ribcage, and the upper chest. After you draw a full, comfortable breath, hold it for a count of three, then let the air out slowly at the same rate and rhythm as the intake. The exhalation order is the exact reverse of the inhalation, in that the air leaves the upper chest, then the ribcage, and finally the abdomen. Allow the abdomen rather than the chest wall to power the breathing process, and try to breathe silently.

Breathe with concentration for a few minutes. Do it now. Settle into a comfortable posture and relax, but don't slump. Sit on a bench or chair with knees uncrossed and feet flat on the floor, or cross-legged on the floor on a cushion, folded towels, or a pillow. I sit on a chair sometimes, or on the floor on a quarter-moon-shaped pillow. The crossed-leg position, with buttocks slightly elevated, is great for smooth breathing and proper posture. Place your hands in one of two positions: the Zen mudra position, which is right hand palm up on the lap, left hand on top of right hand, also palm up, with the balls of the thumbs touching lightly. The alternate hand position is left hand on left thigh, right hand on right thigh, both with palms up, gently touching the thumb of each hand to the index finger. Doing nothing but monitoring your breathing, maintaining proper posture, and using one of the hand positions, you stay alert and focused. You are meditating. Notice as you do this that your mind becomes more tranquil and aware.

MINDFULNESS MEDITATION

The other type of meditation is mindfulness meditation. According to Dr. Joan Borysenko, author of *Inner Peace for Busy People*, mindfulness meditation involves opening your mind's attention to become aware of the continuously passing parade of sensations and feelings, images, thoughts, sounds, smells, and so forth without becoming involved in thinking about them or giving them our judgments. The meditator sits quietly and simply witnesses whatever goes through the mind, not reacting or becoming emotionally involved with thoughts, memories, worries, or images. This helps the meditator gain a calmer, clearer, and less reactive state of mind. Mindfulness meditation can be likened to a wide-angle lens—a broad, sweeping awareness that takes in the entire field of perception without concentrating on any one thing.

Mindfulness is an ancient Buddhist practice that has profound relevance for today, says Kabat-Zinn. Mindfulness has nothing to do with becoming a Buddhist, he points out, but is a way of "waking up and living in harmony with oneself and with the world." Living mindfully is paying complete attention to whatever we're doing, allowing the "mind to be full" of the experience. We are often more asleep than awake to the unique beauty and possibilities of each present moment as it unfolds. We're usually absorbed in anticipating the future—planning strategies to ward off things we don't want to happen and to force outcomes that we do want—or in remembering who did what to whom and why in the past. Such mental gymnastics can leave us exhausted, or at the very least nettled. Most of us spend very little time being aware of the present moment.

The opposite of mindfulness is mindlessness—doing things without thinking, without much feeling, automatically and unconsciously like a robot. Although it is the tendency of our mind to go on automatic pilot, we can also call on our mind to help us awaken to each present moment and use it to advantage. We need to cultivate these moments of mindfulness because they are truly the only moments we have in which to live, grow, feel, love, learn, create, and heal. Coming out of automatic pilot and observing more deeply allows us to feel more connected to what's going on around us and to develop a greater understanding of the order of things. In mindfulness we examine who we are, reevaluate our view of the world and our place in it, and learn how to appreciate the fullness of each moment we are alive.

When you practice mindfulness, you are in touch at all times with yourself and your surroundings, but just as a garden requires tending if you hope to grow flowers and not weeds, mindfulness requires regular cultivation. It doesn't happen all by itself. The beauty of it is that you carry this garden with you wherever you go, wherever you are, whenever you remember to explore it. It is outside of time as well as in it. Kabat-Zinn calls this mind cultivation "wakefulness meditation." You will find that the meditative disciplines, whether they involve mindfulness or concentrative techniques, bring calmness and stability into life.

WHERE TO MEDITATE

It isn't necessary to travel to the Holy Land or the Himalayas to find a good meditation space. Dean Ornish began setting aside a space at home for his meditations when he was an undergraduate in college. "I was living in a one-bedroom apartment," he says, "and I didn't have a room I could use for that purpose. I didn't even have a corner of a room. But I had two closets. One I used for clothing; the other was for meditation." He recommends dedicating some space exclusively to prayer or meditation. Doing so enhances the meditation and makes not only that space but the home around it more sacred.

It's easy to create a personal sacred space. Ornish suggests, "You can put up a picture of a religious or holy person, or someone whose image evokes a sense of calmness or peace and love, or just set up a candle—whatever has the meaning for you of being sacred or inspiring."

A sacred place is where you find tranquility, where you will relish moments of rich solitude. "In your sacred space, things are working in terms of your dynamic and not anybody else's," explains Joseph Campbell. "Your sacred space is where you can find yourself again and again."

For some uplifting and practical material on effective meditation and prayer, I recommend my audio programs, *Wired to Meditate* and *Choose to Live Peacefully*, in addition to my books, *Healthy, Happy & Radiant . . . at Any Age* and *Walking on Air*.

HOW TO BEGIN

I have been a disciplined meditator for the past 35 years, and for 25 years I've been a meditation counselor, conducting workshops and seminars around North America as well as working one-on-one with individuals and families on simple ways to practice meditation to foster health, joy, and peace. So you see, I've benefited from decades of firsthand experience on the efficacy of meditation and how to incorporate it into busy lifestyles. You can learn about my experiences and how to meditate with ease and grace in my audio book, *Wired to Meditate*. Here's a brief summary to get you started:

First, decide where you are going to meditate and create an altar for yourself. It can be decorated with uplifting books, pictures, or objects such as statues, candles, or flowers—anything that makes you feel serene—but keep it simple and clean. For more than 25 years I have set aside a corner of my bedroom as my place of meditation. On my altar (which is really an upside-down wicker basket) I have placed a natural cloth covering and some items that inspire me, including pictures of Jesus and Paramahansa Yogananda, the Bible, Unity's *Daily Word*, a candle, and some fresh flowers. I usually sit on the floor, as I said, on a pillow designed for meditation—but sitting in a chair would be okay, too. Make sure the seat of the chair is parallel to the floor and that your spine is straight. In other words, it's best (sorry to say) not to meditate in your comfortable reclining lounge chair.

Next, pick a regular time to meditate every day. Make it a top priority in your life. Commit yourself to meditating on a regular basis. Some of you may want to think of your meditation session as a daily appointment with the Infinite, and keep that appointment without fail. I devote the early morning before sunrise to meditation, as well as the early evening. This disciplined practice helps me start and end the day on a peaceful, positive note. If you can, choose a quiet time of day for meditating. Earplugs are sometimes helpful.

If you aren't comfortable sitting on the floor, select a chair where you can sit with your spine straight—posture is important. It's mentioned above, but bears repeating: the chair seat should be flat and parallel to the ground. Sitting with your back and neck straight, not supported by the chair's back, will make the energy flow more easily through your spine. Find a position you can sit in fairly comfortably without slumping. Lying down is not recommended because it encourages falling asleep.

As in any physical activity, it is better to begin with brief sessions of meditating and develop a regular practice than it is to start by sitting for hours at a time and then give up in frustration. I recommend starting with ten to 15 minutes once a day. In the beginning it is most important to establish a regular time for meditation and to stick with it. Later you may want to meditate more frequently or for greater lengths of time.

Regardless of the technique you use, you'll find that the mind wanders and the body experiences unusual sensations. Most traditions recommend that you not try to avoid thinking or being distracted. When you realize you are distracted, gently bring your mind back to its object of concentration. Each time the mind wanders and is brought back, your ability to concentrate has been strengthened. Your mind is being trained to respond to you, rather than being allowed to lead you according to its whims. Let's say you have chosen to focus on your breath as you slowly and deeply inhale and exhale. The minute you become aware that you're not focusing on your breath, gently but firmly refocus on it. Through this process of focusing and refocusing on one point, your internal "noise" eventually diminishes; your mind is quieter and your energy level is higher.

Deeper levels of meditation begin after the initial noise and distracting thoughts have been cleared away. Usually, periods of quiet, when it's easy to focus, alternate with periods of unintentional random thinking. As you continue to meditate, the times of easier focus, greater clarity, and inner quiet lengthen. These periods of quiet joyfulness are the first goal of meditation. There is no limit to the depth, energy, and peacefulness that can be achieved in meditation.

Each session of meditation should be continued until a quiet mental state is reached. Don't stop in the middle of a lot of thoughts, when you're having difficulty concentrating. Wait until a time when you are quiet, then stop.

The periods of noise and quiet will alternate as your meditation breaks through layers of thoughts and tension. You will feel renewed if you can stop after reaching any still place; it isn't necessary to reach samadhi (bliss) to have a great meditation.

Even though the goal is absolute quiet, it's important to start your sessions with your energy as high as possible. It's nice to have showered first, or at least to feel awake. The more alert and energized you feel, the easier it will be to focus and meditate. It's also best to meditate on an empty stomach, and definitely not after eating a heavy meal.

Don't be too rigid in your practice. On occasion, find other special places to meditate. I often become immersed in meditation in the outdoors—at the beach, in the mountains, out in the desert, or in a nearby park. I welcome the sounds of nature when I meditate outdoors. Being out in nature encourages mindfulness, helping you to see and hear things more clearly and become one with your surroundings.

NATURE MEDITATION

In Joseph Cornell's book *Listening to Nature*, I learned about a nature meditation he refers to as "stillness meditation." It combines concentrative and mindfulness elements. Here's the technique, which I usually practice while out in nature. It helps to quiet restless thoughts and sometimes brings wonderful calmness.

- First, relax the body: Do this by inhaling and tensing all over—feet, legs, back, arms, neck, face—as much as you possibly can. Then exhale and relax completely. Repeat this several times.
- To practice the technique itself: Observe the natural flow of your breath. Do not control the breath in any way! Simply follow it attentively. Each time you inhale, think "still." Each time you exhale, think "ness." Repeating "still ... ness" with each complete breath helps focus your mind on the present moment and keeps your attention from wandering.
- During the pauses between inhalation and exhalation: Stay in the present moment, calmly observing whatever is in front of you. If thoughts of the past or future disturb your mind, just calmly and patiently bring your attention back to what is before you, and to repeating "still ... ness" with your breathing.

Stillness meditation, explains Cornell, "will help you to become absorbed in natural settings for longer and longer periods. Use it when you want to feel this calmness, indoors or outdoors, with eyes open or closed."

WHITE LIGHT MEDITATION

The following kind of meditation, called White Light meditation, is one that can be done anywhere and is easy for beginners as well as advanced students of meditation.

- Sit in a straight-backed chair with spine erect and feet flat on the floor. (You can also sit cross-legged on the floor if you wish). Fold your hands together in your lap, or hold them in prayer position. Eyes may be open or closed.
- Feel yourself relaxing as you take several long, slow, deep breaths.
- Imagine a beautiful white light glowing from within and completely surrounding you. This is your protection as you open sensitive energy centers, and you can use this with any of your meditations.
- For about ten minutes, gently concentrate on a single idea, picture, or word. Select something that is meaningful, uplifting, and spiritual to you. You might even focus on some peaceful music.
- If your mind wanders from your object of focus, gently bring it back to what you are concentrating on.
- After ten minutes, separate your hands and turn them palms up in your lap. If your eyes have been closed, open them.
- Relax your focus on the object of concentration and shift your mind into neutral.

Remain passive, yet alert, for ten more minutes. Gently observe any thoughts and images that may float by. Just be still and detached, and remain present with whatever you are experiencing.

This twenty minute meditation recharges your energy field and nourishes creativity and tranquility. At other times during the day, allow the same sensation of light to flow from within your being, and let it fill your entire body. It's very easy to do, and it puts you into a meditative state.

If you prefer guided relaxation meditations, I have recorded six different pieces as part of my audio program *Celebrate Life!*, which incorporates music and nature sounds. I also have another meditation in my audio book *Wired to Meditate*.

SPIRITUAL BLESSINGS FROM MEDITATION

The longer any individual practices meditation, the greater the likelihood that his or her goals and efforts will shift toward personal and spiritual growth. As I travel around the country giving talks and meeting people, it delights me to learn how many people are taking responsibility for their health and lives and embracing a holistic program that includes meditation. It's not uncommon for me to hear: "I began meditating to decrease my stress and to feel a sense of control in my life. But as my practice deepens, not only do I feel more relaxed, I also am developing a more open heart—more sensitivity, greater compassion, and less negative judgment toward others."

Many individuals who initially learn meditation for its self-regulatory aspects find that as their practice deepens they are drawn more and more into the realm of the spiritual. Meditation is all about breaking out of the everyday world of tensions and thoughts and finding the place of inner peace, calmness, insight, and enlightenment. It will change your life because it changes you. Find the method or methods that suit you best.

As a part of creating vibrant health, our goal must be to integrate spirituality into every area of our lives. The essence of who we are is pure Spirit; we bring it with us in everything we think, feel, say, and do. An 18-inch journey from your head to your heart keeps you open to Spirit's presence. In other words, jettison judgmental, critical, and the-world-centers-around-me type of thinking in favor of being more tenderhearted, as I wrote about in chapter 3. This takes discipline, courage, and a warrior's strength. It's not for the faint of heart or the weak-minded. In his book, *A Path with Heart*, Jack Kornfield writes from a similar perspective. "We need energy, commitment, and courage not to run from our life nor to cover it over with any philosophy—material or spiritual. We need a warrior's heart that lets us face our lives directly, our pains and limitations, our joys and possibilities. This courage allows us to include every aspect of life in our spiritual practice: our bodies, our families, our society, politics, the Earth's ecology, art, education. Only then can spirituality be truly integrated into our lives."

In her work with many cancer and AIDS patients, Dr. Borysenko has observed that many people are interested in meditation as a way of becoming more attuned to the spiritual dimension of life. She reports that many patients die "healed," in a state of compassionate self-awareness and self-acceptance.

Quiet your mind in meditation to experience the perfect rhythm of the universe. When you go within, jettison negative and judgmental thoughts, and allow yourself the freedom to be at peace by simply meditating and experiencing the oneness of all life, you soon start to find that energy which is blissful and enlightening. If meditation is practiced enough, that quiet mind state will convince you of the oneness and perfection of everything.

Although we may look different on the outside, we are all one in spirit with God and with one another, and we share the same innate spirituality. It's hard to remember this truth in today's tumultuous world. When we watch the TV or read the newspaper, it's easy to forget that we're all made of the same stuff, so much more alike than different. By meditating and following a higher guidance, we can naturally live together in peace and harmony. If we are faced with or witnessing intolerance from others, meditation can give us strength to bless the situation and acknowledge that there is a Divine Power in charge. Obstacles are what we see when we take our eyes off the vision and separate ourselves from one another. Although others may seem worlds apart from us, the acceptance we feel in meditation reminds us that we all look at the same sky, bask in the glow of the same sun, and are blessed by the same intelligence that guides the universe. Meditation helps keep our heart connected to God and our eyes focused on our vision.

THE DIVINE SURRENDER

During my meditation period, I often incorporate visualization, affirmations, and prayer, and most often my prayer involves surrender to the Divine. What is it that I surrender? Negative feelings, negative thoughts, fears, resentments, addictions, and resistance.

Resistance to change is nothing more than

hardening of the attitudes.

Yogananda taught me this prayer of surrender: "Lord, no matter what I'm going through, I love You. I am your child; You are with me always." In that prayer of perfect surrender, we feel our life to be in a Divine embrace, and know that everything is well.

Surrender brings with it gratitude. Gratitude, an overflowing feeling of thanksgiving, is the instant response of the soul touched by awareness of the Divine. Sri Daya Mata, president of the Self-Realization Fellowship, says that with even a momentary awakening to Divine Presence, such joyous freedom bathes our consciousness and provides a blessed release from all the tensions and fears and anxieties that weigh us down in this world. In that wordless praise our whole being pours forth a ceaseless "Thank you! Thank you! Thank you!"

Surrender means letting go, trusting in the forces and principles that are always at work in the universe, and living with spiritual elegance. With surrender comes an inner knowing and contentment. With surrender we can see the perfection of life and accept the paradox that all the suffering in the world is a part of that perfection, as is our own strong desire to help end it. One positive way to surrender is to make a personal commitment to forgive every single person with whom we have ever had any conflict, starting with ourselves. Brook no interference in this process of forgiveness, as it will transform and enrich your life in miraculous ways. Your resplendent Self will shine through and serenity will become your joyful companion.

Choosing to forgive unlocks the gate to healing and health, prosperity and abundance, joy and happiness, and inner peace. Forgiveness is integral to the teachings of Jesus and is also the central teaching of *A Course in Miracles*, a profound set of teachings that I would encourage you to become familiar with. The Course shows how forgiveness can heal our minds, dispel our pain, and ultimately awaken us from the confines of time and space. The core lesson is that fear is an illusion, only love is real, and forgiveness is the vehicle that helps us to release fear. Through forgiveness, miracles occur.

Medical researchers are also coming to the conclusion that an unforgiving nature may be one of the major culprits in human disease. One researcher calls arthritis "bottled hurt." If we condemn, criticize, or resent or if we feel guilty, shameful, or angry toward another, we are only hurting ourselves. And until we practice forgiveness in our lives, the past will continue to repeat itself.

You become linked to another person when you don't offer forgiveness. You also give away your power and create a highly charged, emotionally active connection. But when you forgive, you take back your power and can no longer be controlled by the other person.

Some may say that forgiveness is a sign of weakness. I don't agree with that. It takes strength and courage and a generous spirit to understand that people do not always hurt us because they choose to, but more likely because they couldn't help it or because we were in their way.

People do harm to others when they are in pain and are out of alignment with their Source. If you give back to another person the same pain that person has given you, you are hurting yourself and making it impossible for a miracles to occur.

You can transform any negative emotion into love. While you can't control another person's feelings, you can choose what you want to experience and how you want to be. Let kindness and tenderheartedness be your goal. Jesus tells us to love our enemies.

I understand how difficult this can be, especially when you believe someone has wronged you. Maybe you ask yourself, "How can I forgive what this person has done to me?" The secret is to get yourself out of the way and let Spirit forgive through you. When you choose to live your life more internally, allowing the Infinite to express itself through you, your heart softens and your life changes. Resentments, anger, guilt, and hurt are released. But you can't always release these negative emotions yourself. In my prayer time every day, I ask Spirit to show me how to forgive the past, to forgive others, and to forgive myself.

Make meditation and prayer a top priority in your life. In time, and with disciplined practice, your life will become an expression of meditation and prayer, mindful and concentrated all the time. Meditation and prayer are the medium of miracles. When you meditate and pray, you can't not change. The joy you receive can be continuous.

Some of the prayers I say each day include:

- Make me an instrument of peace and harmlessness.
- I behold the Divine in everyone and everything.

The more you can love everything and everyone and feel gratitude for every moment, the healthier and more balanced your life will be.

> *This is the true joy in life, the being used for a purpose recognized by yourself as a mighty one . . . the being a force of Nature instead of a feverish selfish little clod of ailments and grievances complaining that the world will not devote itself to making you happy.*
> —GEORGE BERNARD SHAW

> *It is one of the most beautiful compensations of this life that no man can sincerely try to help another without helping himself . . . Serve and thou shall be served.*
> —RALPH WALDO EMERSON

CHAPTER 7

Nourish Yourself with Living Foods
I Choose to Support My Own Radiant Health

*Let your food be your medicine . . . let your medicine
be your food.*
—Hippocrates

Food is a love note from God.
—Gabriel Cousens, MD

Last year a man came to me for a consultation. This president
of a major American corporation—we'll call him Arthur—was
impatient, aggressive, sometimes hostile, and unaware of how to
make choices to support his well-being. He routinely put in six or
seven long, pressure-packed days a week at the office or traveling.
He always had to be first, always had to be right, and always had
to be busy with work to feel worthwhile. Playful behavior did
not enter into his lifestyle. As a fancier of rich foods, he put away
vast quantities of cheese, ice cream, steak, butter, processed foods,
and cream sauces. He knew his food was loaded with cholesterol
and fat, but he loved it all the same. As he told me once, when it
came to food he could resist anything but temptation. The most
vigorous exercise he got was shifting gears in one of his expensive
sports cars.

Arthur was usually tired but thought his hot tub and a drink
were all he needed to relax. It wasn't until he began to sink into
a deep depression that his wife urged him to have a medical

checkup, his first in more than five years. Then came the shock: This 45-year-old man discovered he had high blood pressure and serious hardening of the arteries. He was told that if he didn't make some changes in his way of life immediately, he was headed for a heart attack within six months. He was also advised to have quadruple heart bypass surgery.

As providence would have it, the following day a friend of Arthur's, having heard about the doctor's prognosis, recommended that he follow the holistic health regimes and De-Stress Retreat programs detailed in my books, *Health Bliss*, *Recipes for Health Bliss*, *The Healing Power of NatureFoods*, and *Be Healthy-Stay Balanced: 21 Simple Choices to Create More Joy & Less Stress*, as well as my series of booklets on herbs, including *Herbs: Nature's Medicine Chest, Culinary Herbs: Discover the Secrets in Your Spice Rack, Weight Loss: Make it Easy with Herbs*, and *Natural Stress Solutions: Discover Nature's Secret to Inner Calm, Restful Sleep & Newfound Energy*. That's why he sought me out. We worked together on his wellness program. His experiences and adventures over the months since then have been a great inspiration to me, for I had never worked with anyone before who was quite so stressed and desperate, and who led such an unhealthy life. During our first visit he made a choice—he chose to make a commitment to change his life and to be healthy. Today Arthur and his whole family are the picture of health. Recently they participated all together in a 10K run, and the following day they left on a two-week health and fitness vacation.

Vibrant health and happiness are more than just feeling OK, as Arthur learned. They include a quality of life, a joy and radiance that turn each moment every day into a celebration. For most of us, being radiantly healthy is a matter of choice, and the good news is that we can choose to eat in a way that enlivens us physically, emotionally, mentally, and spiritually. I call this approach to food "spiritual nutrition" and it centers on emphasizing live-food cuisine.

It's hard to celebrate life when we're burdened with aches and pains, lethargy, obesity, heart disease, cancer, and other prevalent diseases and ailments of our society. In my decades of work as a holistic lifestyle coach, I have seen thousands of people markedly improve their health and thus enrich their lives through simple dietary changes. My approach to healthful eating is a diet of whole foods, as close as possible to the way Mother Nature has created them. It is this type of diet that restores harmony to the body, mind, and spirit, and replenishes our Life Force. In order to bring a sacred balance into our lives, we must choose foods that not only nourish all the cells of our body, but also feed our souls.

Three of the most incredible and miraculous things about our physical bodies are that they are self-healing, self-purifying, and self-maintaining if we simply fuel them with the living foods they were designed to use by the Creator. All of my books mentioned above go into the specifics of creating the optimum nutrition program and contain loads of recipes that are as easy to make as they are delicious and healthy. Therefore, I will not provide any recipes in this chapter but instead will talk about the specifics of spiritual nutrition. The physical part is the use of fresh, raw, living foods that nourish, cleanse, and alkalinize (change the pH of the blood) the body. They do this through the combined action of their nutritional components: vitamins, minerals, amino acids, liquids, complex carbohydrates, fiber, and especially oxygen and enzymes.

The heart of any living-food diet is fresh fruits and vegetables. Living foods are raw foods not heated above 110 degrees. Driven by mounting scientific evidence, every national health organization, including the National Institutes of Health (NIH), have revised their dietary advice by putting a rainbow of fruits and vegetables front and center, where they belong. Fruits and vegetable are low in calories and high in nutrients—ideal foods for healing, vitality, and weight loss. Nature has color-coded them. A simple way to assure you're getting a healthy variety of nutrients is to enjoy a panoply of colorful foods.

When you look to Nature's treasure chest of foods, especially produce such as fresh fruits and vegetables, you notice an array of colors. Much of the nutritional value in the foods we eat comes from the colors of the food that are teeming with phytonutrients, vitamins, minerals, and enzymes. In fact, quite often the colorful skin of the produce is what provides the most nutritional value—the most bang for your buck.

LIVING FOODS

There is a way to eat that extracts life-sustaining energy from Mother Nature and helps open the subtle energy bodies to the living spirit within them. The more you open your body cells to the Life Force, allowing it to flow through you, the more love, joy, health, happiness, and vitality you will have. You will fill every room you walk into with Light. This is what I mean by spiritual nutrition.

Spiritual nutrition is not a quick fix or a fad diet that depends on and perpetuates addictive, destructive behavior patterns. It contains no prepackaged meals, energy bars, canned drinks, or shots. This new approach to eating introduces your taste buds to exciting natural sensations that are nurturing, balancing, cleansing, rejuvenating, vitalizing, and deeply satisfying. Here are some of the benefits you can look forward to with this way of eating, benefits I've seen from working with thousands of people who embraced spiritual nutrition:

- Easy fat loss
- Increased energy and vitality
- Clearer, more logical thinking
- Increased creativity
- Improved eyesight
- Elimination of pollen and animal allergies
- Increased sexual energy
- Increased resistance to cold and hot weather
- Faster reflexes
- Fresher breath and decreased body odor
- A more positive attitude towards yourself and life
- Deeper connection with the order of things
- Decreased stress
- Increased confidence
- Controlled temper
- Better sense of smell and hearing
- Quick, strong growth of hair and fingernails
- Faster reflexes
- Greater intuitive abilities
- Deeper meditations
- Stronger connections with your angelic guides
- Reconnection with your Higher Self
- And so much more.

Have I your full, undivided attention now?

My interest in living foods began almost 40 years ago, when I was introduced to the Essene movement by my grandmother Fritzie. Jesus and His family were associated with the Essene community. The Essenes were very evolved people who had broken away from the mainstream of Jewish thought several hundred years before the time of Jesus. They were the spiritual heroes of their day, focusing their whole lives on spiritual development and achievement. They were devout lovers of peace and were particularly orderly and clean in their habits. Most important, they were a people who believed in action—in doing rather than talking, and practicing themselves what they then taught to others. They actually lived their philosophy of nonresistance, harmlessness, returning good for evil, and above all, blending the individual spirit with the Spirit of Infinite Love. (For excellent and inspiring reading on the Essene, refer to the book, *Creating Peace by Being Peace: An Essene Sevenfold Path,* by Gabriel Cousens, MD.)

The lives of the Essenes required a discipline and purity of body, mind, and spirit that were beyond the practice of the typical religious person of that time. The Essenes developed self-sufficient communities in a remote desert area in order to make it easier to focus on God. It is thought that Jesus and His parents came from the Essenes, some of whom were also called the Nazarenes, and that they escaped to an Essene community in the desert to avoid the murderous intent of King Herod. Jesus was raised and trained among the Essenes and then went out, like John the Baptist, to preach to the people. As part of their teaching of compassion and love for all life, the Essenes taught vegetarianism. They were said to eat primarily live, or raw, foods and were reported by anthropological historians to live an average of 120 years. In *The Essene Gospel of Peace, Book One*, discovered in 1927 by Dr. Edmond Bordeaux Szekely (who translated the *Essene Gospel of Peace, Books I–IV*), Jesus is quoted as saying:

God commanded your forefathers: "Thou shalt not kill." But their heart was hardened and they killed. Then Moses desired that at least they should not kill men, and he suffered them to kill beasts. And then the heart of your forefathers was hardened yet more, and they killed men and beasts likewise. But I do say to you: Kill neither men nor beasts, nor yet the food which goes into your mouth. For if you eat living (uncooked) food, the same will quicken you, but if you kill your food, the dead food will kill you also.

In the same book, we also find these words of Jesus:

And your bodies become what your foods are. Therefore, eat not anything
which fire, or frost, or water has destroyed.
For burned, frozen and rotted foods will burn, freeze,
and rot your body also.
Be not like the foolish husbandman who sowed in his ground cooked,
frozen, and rotted seeds. And the autumn came, and his fields bore
nothing. And great was his distress.
But be like the husbandman who sowed in his field living seed,
and whose field bore living ears of wheat, paying a hundredfold for the
seeds he planted.
For I tell you truly, live only by the fire of life, and prepare not your foods
with the fire of death, which kills your foods, your bodies,
and your souls also.

Through my decades of research on the Essenes, I have come to
share their aspirations and to see them as my model of excellence.
The Essenes devoted themselves to spiritual evolution, healing,
and service to others—they held a special place in history by living in complete peace and harmony for more than 400 years until
their destruction by the Romans. For more information on them,
you can refer to the many books by Szekely and *Sevenfold Peace*
by Gabriel Cousens, MD. What's germane to this chapter is their
knowledge of the great benefits of living foods.

When you consume living foods, or practice spiritual nutrition, you set in motion the cleansing of the body. At the same
time, you receive an abundant supply of essential, vitalizing Life
Force energy, biologically active enzymes, and other live nutrients
to build and sustain a clean, healthy body. The known constituents of live foods (you can substitute the words "raw," "fresh," or
"uncooked"), and probably other constituents yet unknown, are in
the original life-giving form your body recognizes. They provide

the nutritional conditions necessary to increase the health of the soul as well as the body. You might call them the prerequisite for going beyond mere physical regeneration to physical, mental, emotional, and spiritual resurrection.

From the moment we know our true worth and gain our first spiritual awareness, we naturally become more interested in eating in accordance with God's design and allowing our physical selves to reflect our very highest natures. Health, vitality, balance, longevity, natural beauty, energy, a grateful attitude, empowerment, loving and supportive relationships, right thought, right action, and right living—these are some of the positive natural side effects of spiritual growth. We can unlock an unfailingly loving source of new abilities by choosing to eat more living foods.

In her wonderful book, *Rawsome!*, Brigitte Mars also supports a living foods diet:

The raw path has been used to improve the health of those with arthritis, asthma, high blood pressure, cancer, diabetes, digestive disturbances, menstrual problems, allergies, obesity, psoriasis, skin conditions, heart disease, diverticulitis, weakened immunity, depression, and hormonal imbalances. On a raw diet, degenerative diseases often disappear. The aging process can slow. Bad breath and body odor can go away. Eyes will become brighter and the voice more clear. Skin and muscle tone will improve. Memory and concentration can become sharper. You'll feel better, have more energy, and need less sleep. By following a raw foods diet, you can easily normalize your weight without restricting food intake. Those extra pounds you've been trying to lose will melt away, without your having to go hungry, and your body will maintain its optimal weight for as long as you stay raw.

THE BIOELECTRICITY OF LIVE FOOD

As open-minded as I always aspire to be, I nevertheless appreciate scientific documentation, especially when it comes to nutrition. Scientific studies disclose that the electrical potential of our tissues and cells is a direct indication of their aliveness. What live foods do is enhance the aliveness of our cells, maximizing the electrical potential in and between cells by means of the microcapillary electrical charge. The proper microelectrical potential gives cells the power to rid themselves of toxins and maintain their selective capacity to bring in the appropriate nutrients and oxygen supply. (For some impressive scientific studies and photographs corroborating this, please refer to the book *Conscious Eating* by Gabriel Cousens, MD)

All human tissues and cells are electrically charged; in fact, they work very much like an alkaline battery. Just as an alkaline battery has a positive and a negative pole, a cell has a nucleus and cytoplasm that attract opposite charges: the nucleus is the positive "pole" while the cytoplasm is the negative "pole." As the opposite charges collect in their respective areas, the potential for energy flow in a cell increases. "The greater the energy potential, the healthier the cell," writes Rhio in her terrific book *Hooked on Raw*.

Both an alkaline battery and a human cell rely on chemistry to create their opposite charges, and a living-foods diet replenishes the necessary bioactive alkaline and acid elements to keep cellular energy high and acid waste products low. As I said, the strength of the electrical fields indicates the strength of the cells, and the proper electrical charges in and between cells allow the cells to rid themselves of toxins and bring in the nutrients and oxygen they need for maximum energy. This process is the key to health and longevity. Cells die when the chemistry of the cytoplasm turns acidic and the potential energy drops below a threshold to support this give-and-take life function in the cells. A drop in the electrical potential of the cells is the first step in the disease process. This happens even before laboratory and diagnostic tests can find anything wrong.

Professor Hans Eppinger, chief medical doctor at the First Medical Clinic of the University of Vienna, found that a live-food diet specifically raises the microelectrical potentials throughout the body, increasing the selective capacity of the cells by increasing the electrical potential between tissue cells and capillary cells. His work also established that raw foods significantly improved the intra/extra-cellular excretion of toxins and absorption of nutrients. Additionally, Dr. Eppinger and his colleagues found that live foods were the only foods that could restore the microelectrical potential of the tissue once it had been weakened and the ensuing cellular degeneration had begun to occur.

KIRLIAN PHOTOGRAPHY: SEEING FOOD'S LIFE FORCE

A live-food cuisine, then, is a powerful, natural healing force that gradually restores the microelectrical potential and overall cellular functioning in every cell in our body. I have long found that eating primarily raw foods is a gentle, delicious, nature-oriented, and gradual way to restore health.

Further evidence has been provided by a process known as Kirlian photography, which is the capturing on film of electrical "auras," and electrotherapy. Kirlian photographs by Harry Olfield and Roger Coghill, in their insightful book *The Dark Side of the Brain*, reveal an electroluminescent field surrounding living organisms. Olfield is the world's leading researcher in Kirlian photography. Coghill is a Cambridge scientist. It is believed that what is seen in these photographs is the electrical conductivity of the skin cells as they are influenced by cellular radiations of the rest of the cells of the body. Olfield and Coghill feel that these electrical fields actually maintain the integrity of the biological system. They hypothesize, as I do, that human beings and all living organisms are ultimately made up of patterns of resonant energy. The basic molecular structure of each cell is guided by DNA, which acts as a resonant receiver of the different resonant frequencies of the body and also as a transmitter of its own specific resonant frequency. The stronger the resonant frequency of the cell, the healthier it is and the stronger its natural radiation field is. In other words, the electroluminescence of the cells is a measure of their Life Force. Kirlian photography, by recording this electroluminescence, shows the electrical potential and therefore the living energy of each cell.

By using this system, Olfield and Coghill were able to document how the Life Force of individuals and foods is affected by various conditions. The two authors selected 12 average people on what they called an "everyday" diet. Most of the subjects initially showed very weak energy fields in the Kirlian photographs. After these same people were fed a 24-hour "junk food" diet consisting entirely of processed food with the usual chemicals, preservatives, and food colorings, the photographs revealed the absence of any electroluminescent energy at all. In contrast, they showed a picture of a man who had been living on whole foods for 40 years. The difference between his highly charged and visible field and the absence of any field in the junk food photographs was dramatic. The man was in peak physical condition, stating that even common colds had been no problem since he'd begun his health diet so many years before. If you can find a copy of this fascinating book, you'll marvel at the Kirlian photographs and will be motivated to improve your diet!

Another photographic comparison the authors made was of the electroluminescence of a cabbage, first raw (live) and then after being cooked in a pressure cooker for ten minutes. The cabbage when it was fresh and alive had a significantly brighter, larger electroluminescent field than when it was cooked. Carrying the comparative process still farther, they applied the Kirlian technology to assessing the effect of different storage techniques and different processing methods on foods. They found that the natural, healthy radiation of the food varied according to the cooking method. Assessing the healthfulness of food processing by the amount of radiation that appeared, from the least damaging to the most, the photographs showed:

1. No cooking (raw)
2. Wok cooking
3. Steaming
4. Microwave cooking
5. Pressure cooking and boiling
6. Deep frying
7. Barbecue and grilling
8. Oven baking

The results for storage methods, again starting from the highest remaining natural radiation, were:

1. Fresh raw food showed the most energy by a significant margin.
2. Raw food stored in the refrigerator for four hours or less was next highest.
3. Freeze-drying left 75 percent of the original energy.
4. Freezing left 30 percent of the original energy.
5. Gamma radiation left almost no natural radiation and completely obliterated the radiation of avocados.

THE BIOPHYSICS OF LIVING FOODS

In the aforementioned *Conscious Eating*, Dr. Cousens addresses the new scientific models developed by the brilliant minds in submolecular biology and quantum physics, which have made it possible to develop corresponding scientific models in the biophysics of nutrition. This expanded conceptual understanding helps us better understand the importance of living foods.

Nobel laureate Dr. Szent Gyorgyi describes the essential life process as a little electrical current sent to us by sunshine. He is referring to highly charged single electrons that transfer their energy to our own submolecular patterns without changing our molecular structure. These wandering sunlight electrons belong to the electron clouds of the submolecular world described by quantum mechanics. These quantum physics models, happily for plant eaters, begin to validate our more intuitive model of vegetarian food as condensed sunlight energy, which is then transferred to our human organism.

To see how it might work, consider that living foods get their electrical charges from the highly charged electrons sent to us by the sun. The foods condense the sunlight energy and feed it to our body's cells. Researchers in this field believe that the condensed electrical energy we take in has the ability to awaken relatively inert molecules in our system, by either taking an electron from them or giving them one. That's why the high electrical potential of living foods is an important factor in their healing power. In essence, by restoring the electrical potential of the cells, raw foods rejuvenate the Life Force and health of the organism.

John Douglass, MD, PhD, of the Kaiser Permanente Hospital in Los Angeles, has investigated the process of revitalizing molecules by the adding or subtracting of electrons. This high-energy electron transfer ability is described as the "high redox potential" of a particular molecule. Vitamin C has this high redox potential, and so do raw foods. Dr. Douglass believes the high redox potential of raw foods, which is destroyed by cooking, is an important factor in their healing power.

Cousens reports other fascinating work by a German researcher, Johanna Budwig, on the interaction of fatty acid and sunlight. Dr. Budwig feels that a particular sun electron, called the biotron, is involved in the production of cellular energy and that the biotron is absorbed directly into the brain. Some scientists have theorized that as much as one-third of our energy comes into our system directly from the sun via the biotron.

Through his own extensive research, Cousens has found that the sunlight energy, when it is transferred to us indirectly through our food, is almost completely lost if the transfer of plant food nutrients is secondhand, by way of animal food. Even in vegetarian food, the Kirlian photography studies suggest that sunlight energy is significantly lost if the bioelectric resonant energy patterns are disrupted by cooking or processing. Thinking of food and the human body in terms of bioelectric energy, then, we have to conclude that foods in their live state pass energy from the sun directly and maximally to us.

Plants store the energy for us in their work of photosynthesis. Put another way, plants release their stored light to us. This is one of the great secret stories of live foods. Our biological lives and health are dependent on the electromagnetic radiation of the sunlight. This bioelectric radiation stored in the plants, as nature's gift to us, is lost or greatly diminished when live foods are cooked, irradiated, or even stored for more than a few days. If we increase the bioelectrical energy in our cells, by eating food as close as possible to its growing state, we increase our health, vitality, and longevity.

IN SUPPORT OF LIVE FOOD

Francis M. Pottenger, Jr., MD, performed some of the earliest and most significant studies of live food. I discovered his work when I was at UCLA, writing my Masters thesis on "The Effects of Diet and Exercise on Health and Longevity." One report, which appeared in the *American Journal of Orthodontics and Oral Surgery* in 1946, detailed the results of a ten-year study of 600 cats. The results showed the destructive effect of cooked foods (diet-deficient foods) and the health-promoting effects of raw food (optimum-diet foods) across generations.

Pottenger observed that cats on a raw-food diet were healthy and reproduced normally. They were fed a diet of 2/3 raw meat, 1/3 raw milk, and cod liver oil. The cats given cooked-food diets including meat, pasteurized milk, evaporated milk or sweetened condensed milk showed marked physical degeneration and reproductive breakdown. This degeneration increased with each generation and was most severe in the group that was fed sweetened milk. If the cats were fed raw meat, but with it pasteurized milk instead of raw milk, the degeneration progressed. Kittens in the third generation on the cooked diets failed to survive six months.

Here are some other dramatic effects that appeared in the study: skin diseases and allergies increased from an incidence of 5 percent in normal cats to more than 90 percent in the third generation of cats fed the cooked-food diets. Susceptibility to infections rose markedly (likely due to immune deficiency syndromes), and severe osteoporosis was universal. Mortality was high.

All of the cats fed cooked diets suffered from most of the degenerative diseases encountered in human medicine, including cancers of all kinds. Change was evident not only in the immediate generation, but also as a "germ-plasma injury" passed on to each new generation, making the offspring even less resistant to disease. If the cats' natural diet—the fresh, uncooked diet—was reintroduced to the second generation of cats, it took four generations on the raw diet to produce healthy cats once again. If the uncooked diet was reintroduced in the third generation, the following generations of cats never did achieve normal health.

To finish the experiment, Dr. Pottenger studied plants fertilized by manure from the two groups of cats. The plants with the raw-food manure grew excellently. The plants fed the cooked-food manure were weak and struggled to survive, highlighting the lack of any life-giving features in the cooked-food diet.

Whether we're talking about animals or humans, the idea that the body can easily digest and assimilate cooked food may prove to be one of the most harmful assumptions of science. From over three decades of research on nutrition and holistic living, I have no doubt that cooking reduces vitamin and mineral availability; destroys enzymes, natural plant hormones, and oxygen; promotes acid accumulation in the body; interferes with thorough digestion; and weakens the immune system and the bioactive electrical charge of the body's tissues and cells. It also weakens the power of naturally occurring antioxidants. In short, cooking is largely responsible for the toxic dump sites we've created within our bodies. Living foods clean up these dump sites: they cleanse clogged systems, restore radiant health and vitality to all the body cells, and give us personal control over our health and longevity. These are just a few facts of living foods. Let's take a brief look at how live foods boost immunity and increase enzymes.

HOW LIVING FOODS BOOST IMMUNITY

In 1930, research by Paul Kouchakoff, MD, a Swiss physician, showed that every time we eat cooked foods, we get an increase of white blood cells in our blood stream, referred to as "leucocytosis." Repeated leucocytosis following every meal overstimulates the immune system three or four times a day: definitely an ongoing stress on the system. Kouchakoff found that when subjects started a meal with raw foods that equaled more than half of the meal, they were able to have some cooked foods without experiencing leucocytosis. In other words, choose to make at least 50 percent of each meal living food!

Another way raw food helps boost the immune system is that it keeps us healthy with its "anti-free radical" enzymes, cleansing properties, and physical and energetic enhancement of our total biological organism. Research at the Linus Pauling Institute showed that a raw-food diet in mice had the same cancer-preventing properties as high doses of vitamin C. In my own counseling work, I have observed that my clients who have been on an 85 percent or more live-food diet for six months to two years have significantly stronger immune systems than the general population and get significantly fewer colds and flus than they did previously.

ENZYME POWER

If you look up the definition of the word "enzyme" in a dictionary, you'll probably find something like this: "A protein functioning as a biochemical catalyst in a living organism." Sounds simple enough if you're a chemist, but it doesn't begin to describe the incredible complexity of biochemical reactions that take place in the human body.

Many people consider pioneering author of *Food Enzymes for Health and Longevity*, Dr. Edward Howell, the father of food enzyme research in this century. According to Howell, enzymes are not only chemical protein complexes but also bioenergy reservoirs. Because they are large molecules, enzymes are designed to facilitate certain reactions in the body. Each organ has its own set of enzymes. There are three main types: metabolic enzymes, which activate all our metabolic processes; digestive enzymes, for the digestion of food; and a category called food enzymes, which are present in all live foods and serve to activate the digestion of those specific foods in which they occur. Live foods contain a variety of metabolic enzymes as well, and all are essential to the functioning of our bodies.

Of the 1,300-plus enzymes that have so far been identified in the human body, about 24 are digestive enzymes. These fit into three primary categories: proteases digest proteins, amylases digest carbohydrates, and lipases digest fats. Mother Nature contributes to our supply by adding food enzymes to each living food in nature, which come in the exact ratio of the proteases, amylases, and lipases required for the digestion of that particular food. Avocados and nuts, for example, contain naturally-occurring lipase, while oats have a high amount of amylase, or starch-digesting enzyme. The contribution of food enzymes to the digestive process is extremely important to overall digestive function and is too often overlooked.

Shirley was a poignant example of enzyme deficiency. Like many clients who come to me anxious to shed weight, Shirley could never seem to lose any fat. I put her on a well-rounded exercise program, improved her diet from all cooked to some raw food (initially, she was only willing to add in about 20 percent raw food), and encouraged her to drink more water, get more sleep, and reduce the stress in her life. But nothing seemed to help. Discouraged, she was willing to try my recommendation of 85 percent to 15 percent ratio of raw to cooked food, plus the addition of an enzyme supplement to help break down, absorb, and assimilate food easier. She was amazed: for the first time in her life, her extra weight began to decrease. I've seen this occur over and over again and am now a great believer in digestive enzyme supplementation, especially as people get older (digestive enzymes decrease with age) or if they eat a lot of cooked foods.

Research supports my treatment: a doctor at Tufts Medical School found that 100 percent of the cases of obesity he studied had lipase deficiencies! The implication was that they had a decreased ability to assimilate fat, so that it ended up being stored as fatty tissue instead of being broken down and used or eliminated.

Besides being enzyme-deprived, cooked food also seems to stimulate the craving for more food in general, according to Vibrance (*www.livingnutrition.com*), a magazine dedicated to healthy foods and balanced living. The organs are not receiving the nutrients they would normally get in uncooked food, so the body naturally craves more nutrients, and this can translate into an uncontrollable appetite and lack of willpower. Farmers have known for a long time that if you give raw potatoes to hogs they do not gain weight, but if you give them cooked potatoes they do. In my practice, I often see people lose weight easily and effortlessly when they merely add more raw food to their diet. Many times the addition of raw food is all that is needed.

DANIELLE'S STORY: CHANGE YOUR DIET, CHANGE YOUR LIFE

For those of you who haven't read the sections of my books, *Health Bliss* and *Recipes for Health Bliss,* where I wrote about one of my clients, Danielle, here's a brief summary of her story. Danielle is a great example of how changing our diet and adding more raw foods can not only assist with weight loss but also improve every aspect of family life and self-esteem. A married woman with three children ages five, eight, and eleven, Danielle initially came to me for motivation and help in losing some fat, toning up her body, and increasing her energy. As a first step, I asked her to keep a seven-day food diary and record exactly what and when she ate. Like all my new clients, she was instructed not to eat differently simply because I would be looking at the list; she had to be honest and write down everything, because there's no other way to make a true evaluation.

When I received her food diary, it was quite apparent why she had gained almost 30 pounds in a year and always felt ener-vated. Her diet was about 60 percent fat, the carbohydrates she consumed were almost all refined, she usually skipped breakfast because she was too busy getting the kids ready for school, and she always ate late at night. Her diary came straight out of my "encyclopedia of deleterious habits"! She rarely included raw foods in her diet or her family's, explaining that it took too long to chew the food and she didn't have time. Danielle also noted that her kids disliked raw foods, so only on rare occasions did she have a few fruits and vegetables in the house.

As I inquired more about her family life, routines, eating habits, and so on, I learned that each of her children was on the heavy side. The oldest girl was starting to be ridiculed in school because of her size. Not surprisingly, Danielle told me that her husband also needed to lose about 40 pounds. His blood pressure, cholesterol, and triglycerides were much too high and his doctor had suggested that he go on a diet. I told Danielle that no diet was necessary. Her family needed a health makeover, and I assured her that she had come to the right person for guidance.

My initial evaluation of how they ate and lived led me to suggest something very out of the ordinary. Knowing that they had a large house with a guest room next to the kitchen, I asked if I could stay with them from Thursday through Saturday night. I wanted to experience their lifestyle as a family, to see how they lived at home, when and what they ate, and how they spent their time when not eating in order to coach them toward a healthier way of living. Yes, I brought most of my own food, and I simply observed like a butterfly on the wall (I prefer butterflies to flies) and took lots of notes. I had Danielle's permission, when they were out of the house, to look through their pantry and refrigerator and all their kitchen cupboards. Sure enough, I found hardly any fresh, whole foods.

At mealtime, everyone salted the food before tasting it, and their dining table was never without canned sodas or processed fruit juices, butter, sour cream, and mounds of cheese. All five family members ate their meals quickly, without much conversation and without putting the utensils down between bites. Much overeating may be unintentional, since many popular foods contain hidden sugar and oils put there to stimulate the taste buds, and this was definitely the case with Danielle's family.

With Danielle's consent, I made a clean sweep of her kitchen. The rest of her family went along, although they were far from enthusiastic. I removed all refined carbohydrates, including pasta, white rice, low-fiber cereals, pancake and cookie mixes, white breads, and bagels, and gave them to a homeless shelter. (There are ways to make deleterious foods healthier. So whenever I take less-than-optimal food to a shelter, I encourage them to add fiber, fruit, greens, or whatever they have available to these foods so that the recipients will receive some nutrients. With more nutrients in their diet, the homeless will have more energy and become more positive and hopeful.) I replaced these with high-fiber breads and whole grains. I also rid their kitchen of margarine, mayonnaise, and vegetable shortenings and oils. Next I gave away all the whole milk and cheese products. Those high-fat, calorie-loaded cheese slices provide between 80 and 140 calories per one-ounce slice, depending on the fat content. I replaced the whole milk with non-fat and also introduced them to nut and seed milks, which are easy to make; it turned out that they all loved the vanilla-flavored almond and cashew nut milk after about two weeks of adapting to the new taste, and eventually they gave up dairy milk.

I took the entire family to the nearest health food store, showed them all the healthy alternatives such as veggie burgers and whole-grain pastas and, to the amazement of all of them, let them experience the produce section of the store. They were enthralled by all the colors and varieties of fruits and vegetables, many of which they had never seen before. We started with some of the most familiar— apples, oranges, pears, grapes, bananas, and strawberries.

In place of sodas and other canned drinks, I taught them how to make their own juice. The kids loved juicing and actually wanted to take it over as their daily job. Of course I encouraged them to start drinking more water. Danielle's husband confessed to me secretly that he couldn't remember having more than about six glasses of water weekly. When I told him that I drink almost 100 ounces of pure water every day, he almost collapsed in shock.

Yes, it took about one month for the family to adjust their taste buds to the new flavors, textures, and colors of their foods. They basically switched from a white and beige diet to a banquet of rainbow colors. Almost half their diet was now raw foods, with an abundance of fresh fruits and vegetables. When you fill up on these salutary foods, you nourish your body and actually lose much of your desire for junk or other processed foods.

After several private cooking (and un-cooking) lessons with me, Danielle found it wasn't so hard to cook healthier meals. As a result of eating more fiber and more nutritious foods, everyone in the family lost weight and had more energy and balanced moods as well as a greater sense of well-being that resulted in more positive attitudes all around. I encouraged them all to be more active instead of hanging out in front of televisions or computers most nights and weekends, and their higher activity resulted in sounder sleep for everyone. Danielle's oldest daughter lost weight and joined an after-school sports team, which ended the ridicule and helped her self-esteem soar.

It's truly remarkable how making a few basic changes in one's diet can profoundly affect every area of life. The change this family had the hardest time with initially, but which ultimately turned out to be the most fun, was the one day each week of raw food. I suggested they not pick a weekend day or a Monday but rather a Tuesday, Wednesday, or Thursday. They selected Thursday and from morning through evening ate only living foods—lots of fruits and vegetables, salads, and a variety of other fun foods including nut butters, sprouts, sauces, soups—even cookies and other desserts. It takes literally a few seconds to make raw fruit, vegetable and even squash or bean soups that are as delicious to eat as they are pleasing to the eye. All you need is a good blender and some terrific recipes. For example, blend together two cups of fresh carrot juice, one pitted avocado, some cilantro and other seasoning of choice and you have a delicious fresh creamy carrot soup. You can warm it if you like, but it's wonderful at room temperature. Or you can blend together three tomatoes, one cucumber, 1/2 avocado, 1/4 cup raw cashews, one red bell pepper, and a pinch of Celtic Sea Salt and you'll have a mouth-watering, nutritious soup. Finally, blend any of your favorite melons (separately or together) with some freshly pressed ginger for a zingy fruit soup. (See my other books for more delicious and easy-to-prepare recipes.) The family came to appreciate Danielle's gift for experimenting and creating new meals with only nutritious raw foods. A few weeks into their new health regime, they started having friends over for meals to sample their delicious "health nut food" and even frequented a local restaurant with live-food cuisine!

Even though you may not be eager to overhaul your entire food program, you can at least start by adding more raw enzyme-rich fruits and vegetables to your diet. I recommend the following regime to my clients and friends. Begin by making at least 50 percent of your diet raw each and every day. On Mondays, eat raw foods all day until dinner (with the cooked food coming only at the end of the evening meal), and on Thursdays, raw foods all day including dinner. This simple program will assist you to bring more living foods into your diet by spacing them out over the week. You'll feel lighter and more energetic immediately simply from eating more uncooked foods.

Enzymes are particularly sensitive to the molecular destruction caused by cooking. Unfortunately, each of us is given only a finite supply of enzyme energy at birth, which must serve to keep every body system in working order throughout its lifetime. The only other source of enzymes we have is the food we eat (or supplements)—but in food cooked above 118 Fahrenheit all the enzymes are killed! So what happens if we make big enzyme withdrawals, as we all do when we catch a virus, do something physically strenuous, face an emotional crisis, breathe unclean air, or get extremely angry or tired, and then compound the problem by eating cooked and processed foods? The balance in our enzyme account can drop dangerously low, and if it's not replenished, the body faces enzyme bankruptcy.

When we make severe demands on any system, including the digestive system, the body puts out an emergency call to enzymes throughout the body. According to Dr. Brian Clement, co-director of the Hippocrates Health Institute in West Palm Beach, Florida, the body will steal enzymes from glands, muscles, nerves, and blood to help in the demanding digestive process. Eventually there is a deficiency of enzymes in those areas, and this, many scientists throughout the world believe, is the real cause of various allergies and diseases. Howell has said that enzyme shortages are commonly seen in a number of chronic illnesses such as allergies, skin disorders, obesity, heart disease, and certain types of cancer, as well as in aging. As a matter of interest, all the people I know who eat most of their diet raw look ten to 20 years younger than their age!

The healing power of enzymes is absolute and proven. Almost every regulatory system in our body depends on enzymes and suffers from their depletion: coagulation, wound healing, and tissue regeneration, to name just a few. The enzyme account throughout the body is replenished by the living foods we eat because the enzymes are absorbed into the blood to reestablish normal blood-serum enzyme levels. To track the whole-body value of an enzyme-rich diet, researchers have tagged enzyme supplements with radioactive dye and traced them through the digestive tract. They discovered that the tagged enzymes could be found in the liver, spleen, kidneys, heart, lungs, duodenum, and bladder/urine.

Eating raw foods is the single most positive thing you can do to preserve and replenish your enzymes and maximize your health. The rest of Mother Nature's children do not cook their food. It is a striking fact that all other species, without exception, eat their foods raw, whereas the overwhelming majority of humans do not. Animals in the wild do not suffer from the same chronic degenerative diseases as do humans and their domesticated animals. When wild animals are fed cooked foods, they, too, begin to suffer chronic diseases.

LIVING FOODS THAT CLEANSE, HEAL, AND REJUVENATE

The evidence is indisputable. Around the world, studies are corroborating the benefits of eating more fresh, raw fruit and vegetables. Here are just a few of the facts:

- The risks of common forms of cancer are reduced by 50 percent in countries where about a pound of fruits and vegetables per person are eaten each day.
- Virtually every disease of aging—including heart disease, diabetes, and many common forms of cancer such as breast cancer and prostate cancer—results from damage to DNA, which can be prevented by the substances found in fruits and vegetables.
- 80 to 90 percent of all cancers are not inherited but begin with the defects in DNA resulting from the accumulated damage of a lifetime—damage that could be prevented by increasing fruit and vegetable intake.

Eating raw foods is the single most positive thing

you can do to preserve and replenish your enzymes and

maximize your health.

These are only a few of the facts I garnered from the excellent book *What Color Is Your Diet ?* by David Heber, MD, PhD, head of the UCLA Center for Human Nutrition. He says most Americans eat far too few foods with any color in them. Studies show that the average total intake of fruits and vegetables is about three servings daily, with a serving consisting of a half-cup of cooked vegetables, a cup of raw vegetables, or a piece of fruit. If those three servings are iceberg lettuce, French fries, and a little ketchup for color, you are in big trouble! Heber writes:

Eating is a pleasure, and we have voted with our dollars for a beige diet of French fries, burgers, and cheese. The only problem with the diet we love is that it doesn't fit our genes, which evolved over eons in a plant-based, hunter-gatherer diet with half the fat, no dairy products, no processed foods, no refined sugars, no alcohol, and no tobacco. Our closest animal relatives, gorillas and chimpanzees, choose a richly diverse selection of plant foods based on color, size, texture, and taste. Today, in places such as New Guinea, we can still find hunter-gatherer populations who eat more than eight hundred varieties of plant foods.

Adding foods is easier than taking them away, and the simple addition to our diet of fruits and vegetables will help protect the genes from being damaged.

Another reason for introducing more diversity into our diets is that different foods provide different plant chemicals, known as phytochemicals. Phytochemicals ("phyto" comes from the Greek word meaning plant) are components within natural food that have been proven to ward off disease and heal the body.

There are thousands of phytochemicals found in plant foods like fruits, vegetables, whole grains, legumes, nuts, and seeds. Here are just a few of the more commonly known, their food sources, and what science tells us about their salubrious function.

- Lycopene—(pink grapefruit, watermelon, and especially tomatoes; for lycopene to be absorbed from the tomatoes, it must be consumed with some fat) Decreases the risk of prostate cancer, probably by reducing DNA damage from oxidation of cells; may also decrease other cancers in women.
- Indoles—(cruciferous vegetables such as broccoli, cabbage, and cauliflower) Reduce the risk of breast cancer by helping the body convert a potentially harmful form of estrogen into a harmless form.

- Isoflavones, also known as phyto-estrogens—(soy beans and dried beans) Reduce the risk of breast and ovarian cancer and osteoporosis; also relieve hot flashes.
- Lutein and zeaxanthin, found together in foods—(yellow, orange, and dark green leafy vegetables) Reduce the risk of macular degeneration, the leading cause of blindness in older people.
- Allyl sulfides—(garlic, onions, leeks, chives) Reduce cancer risk by helping to neutralize carcinogens; also may interfere with reproduction of tumor cells.
- Flavonoids—(apples, celery, cranberries, grapes, black and green tea, onions) Reduce the risk of heart disease by decreasing oxidation of LDL cholesterol.
- Ellagic acid—(strawberries, raspberries, grapes) Protects against carcinogens found in tobacco and environmental pollutants.
- Terpenes—(citrus fruits) Block development of cancer tumors (tamoxifen and taxol, which are used to treat breast cancer, are both terpenes).
- Saponins—(soybeans and other dried beans, quinoa, cherries) Prevent cancer cells from multiplying.
- Isothiocyanates—(cruciferous vegetables such as broccoli, cabbage, and cauliflower) Trigger the formation of enzymes that could prevent carcinogens from damaging DNA.

EATING FOR BODY AND SOUL

Before I end this section on the benefits of eating living foods, I'd like to touch on my personal nutritional regime and the spiritual changes that have come from eating raw foods. I could write an entire book on this topic, but I'll put it in a nutshell for you. For the past 35 years I've been a vegetarian, and a vegan for 15 years, which means I don't eat any animal products, including dairy and eggs. For 20 years I have emphasized live-food cuisine. I eat between 75 to 100 percent of my diet raw, but the percentage varies according to the seasons and my body's needs. For example, every summer I set aside a 40-day period when I follow a 100 percent live-food diet. During springtime and fall, I eat 90-100 percent of my diet raw. In the winter months, when it's colder, I may go to 75-100 percent raw food. In addition, I do a short fresh juice fast with each change of season—more as a spiritual discipline these days than to cleanse and detoxify my body, since my diet contains very few impurities. I also do a longer fresh juice fast every couple of years in the summer.

At first it was difficult to eat more raw foods because my body was accustomed to cooked food and the associated addictive processes. In other words, for many people, cooked foods, especially low nutrient-dense refined foods made with white sugar and white flour and dairy, meat, and other animal products can become addicting. You start to eat them and even though you're not hungry, you want to keep eating more of them. Part of the reason is because your body is never satisfied nutritionally and it craves more food to ensure you're getting all of the nutrients you need. But after a short while—about three weeks—of eating primaily raw food, I started to notice exciting changes in my body and appearance. I had more energy and felt better about myself and more empowered overall. My skin became softer and more youthful. My aches and pains vanished, and my attitude about life became more positive. I felt lighter in every way.

I've always noticed that when my emotional energy is positive, I find it easy to take good care of myself and eat "well." Then, when I am upset or stressed and my emotional energy drops, I begin to crave white sugar or white flour products like pasta or other addictive nonfoods. I bet you've experienced the same thing. I believe we actually seek out food that matches our lowered energy state, as if we are ingesting dead food to match a sort of emotional "dead space" within. When we eat the typical American acid-producing diet of cooked food, without lots of fresh raw fruits and veggies, it inhibits the flow of electrical energy. We experience lethargy, depression, and other challenging emotions, as well as low energy. It's a vicious circle that we can break out of simply by eating more live foods.

As I became more conscious of how the food I ate affected my body, emotions, mind, and spiritual life, I began to understand how what we eat can directly affect the Earth's ecology and the degree of peace we have on this planet. This is what conscious eating and spiritual nutrition are all about.

Other noticeable changes started to happen when the percentage of raw food in my diet reached 85 or more. Doubt, fear, anger, loss of faith, guilt, and ego fell away as I fine-tuned my physical being with this sun-food diet. Raw foods actually change the vibrational rate of the cells and body and we become better receivers of higher energy—the higher energy of your inner Light (or Love). On raw foods, my meditations became deeper and more profound and I felt a deeper level of peace than ever before.

The typical American acid-producing diet of cooked food, without lots of fresh raw fruits and veggies, inhibits the flow of electrical energy. Eating this way, we experience lethargy, depression, and other challenging emotions. It's a vicious circle that we can break out of simply by eating more live foods.

Connecting with the Light of your being, just like conscious eating and spiritual nutrition, is not some far-off goal to be reached someday. In fact, it is not the goal at all, but merely the starting point of a wonderful journey toward your highest spiritual goals. What's important to realize is that you start the minute you adopt a more living-foods diet. It may seem like a big effort, but as you go along your life will feel less encumbered, not more.

THE NUTS AND ETCETERAS OF HEALTHY EATING

One of my clients, Rebecca, is married with four children. Mealtime, she told me, was fraught with more conflict and frustration than pleasure and relaxation. I visited her home for dinner one evening so I could experience her dilemma firsthand. All six family members had different food preferences, and all the food was cooked. During our follow-up counseling session, I suggested that she make a centerpiece out of a large plate of cut-up raw vegetables in a variety of colors—very appealing to both kids and adults. I recommended a large salad with a base of dark leafy greens, such as romaine and baby leaf spinach, along with a variety of colorful chopped vegetables. I also gave her a few ideas for dressings that kids love. Finally, I suggested that she always offer a bowl of steamed vegetables with three or four different colors. One of my favorite combinations is steamed broccoli, baby carrots, yellow squash, and red cabbage. The colors are so beautiful: bright green (especially if the broccoli is not overcooked), orange, yellow, and deep purple. Three to four vegetables make a meal much more filling. And it's amazing how even people who "hate" vegetables will eat them when topped with a delicious sauce, so I referred her to those recipes in my books.

I was so happy to hear Rebecca say, "It's not a lot of work, because I choose vegetables that are simple to prepare, or I buy them ready-to-cook from the supermarket or salad bar." To her delight and surprise, her entire family started eating more vegetables and, because of the natural fiber volume, they had less appetite for processed and junk foods. They found, just as you will, that as your system becomes cleansed and detoxified by the addition of more live foods, you start to lose even your desire for junk food.

As you proceed to make your diet more colorful with raw fruits and vegetables, you will be including more of the delicious raw foods—sprouted seeds, grains, legumes, a limited amount of nuts and seeds (one ounce a day because of their high fat content, if fat loss is desired), and other plant-based foods. I couldn't possibly list them all, but I encourage you to visit your local natural food store and supermarket. Whenever possible, buy organically grown food. If you don't live near a natural food store or farm stand or have access to a garden or a farmer's market in your neighborhood, ask the produce manager at your local supermarket to bring in organic foods. The more we ask for higher-quality food, the more we'll see it in our stores.

To fill in gaps that may exist, even in the healthiest diet, some nutritional supplements may be helpful. On my website, *www.SusanSmithJones.com*, click on Favorite Products, and you see that I recommend some of my favorites.

In my three-book series, *Health Bliss, Recipes for Health Bliss*, and *The Healing Power of NatureFoods*, I urge you to include at least seven to twelve servings of fresh fruits and vegetables in your daily diet, and I provide over 100 suggestions on the best foods to eat. This is not hard if you eat two salads daily and some fresh fruit as your snacks. These foods are the heart of my diet because they provide the richest source of vitamins, minerals, enzymes, antioxidants, fiber, phytochemicals, and all-around health-promoting substances. I eat at least twelve servings a day (Three to four servings of fruit and twelve or so servings of vegetables), because I always have a couple of salads with different vegetables each time. They always include homegrown sprouts, lots of greens (which are rich in chlorophyll—a detoxifying, rejuvenating green substance in plant foods), perhaps a few nuts and seeds, and delicious homemade dressings. Then I'll add other plant-based foods to round out my fruit and vegetable meals.

Here are a few suggestions on how to eat better to live longer.

- Emphasize colorful plant-based foods, starting with at least 50 percent of your diet raw, living foods. Build up to 75 percent or more, after the first year.
- Eat a variety of colorful fruits and vegetables, at least seven to twelve servings daily.
- Eat less fat and take what fat you do consume from whole foods, such as avocado, nuts and seeds, flax seed and oil, etc.
- Stop dieting and quit yo-yoing with your weight.
- Eat three main meals every day, with two or three snacks.
- Have your largest meal at lunch rather than dinner.
- Don't eat two to three hours before bedtime with the exception of something light and easy-to-digest, such as freshly-made vegetable juice, tea, or a piece of fruit.
- If you can't stop with just one, don't drink alcohol before or after meals. Better yet, don't drink at all.
- Drink an 8-ounce glass of fresh vegetable (with carrot) juice daily.
- Don't overeat. Studies reveal that habitual under-eating promotes healing, rejuvenation, and longevity.
- Drink at least eight large glasses of pure water daily.
- Four times a year, with each season, conduct your own detox-rejuvenation retreat by eating only raw, plant-based foods. You'll look and feel years younger. (In my books, I discuss the importance of keeping your body detoxified and provide the easy steps on how to do it.)
- Eat slowly and chew your food well.
- Don't use mealtime to discuss problems. Make it as pleasant and positive as possible.
- Be grateful for your miraculous body and give thanks for your food and meals.
- Eat to live, don't live to eat.
- Make health a top priority in your life and show by your daily food choices that you have high self-esteem and self-respect.
- Stay centered in Spirit, choose to be happy, and love your life—especially when you're preparing and eating Mother Nature's food!

One way to make sure your spirit is nourished is to create a beautiful, serene setting in which to eat. There are five elements that can contribute to the ambiance of your dining area, as well as the rest of your home.

1. Lighting—candles and dimmer switches help create a peaceful, harmonious environment.
2. Sound—I always have the sound of a flowing fountain in my home. It helps foster balance and peace when eating which, in turn, promotes good digestion. Small table fountains can be heard in several rooms at once.
3. Texture—Select placemats, napkins, and dinnerware that bring you joy and pleasure. Remember, dining should be a pleasurable experience.
4. Color—From the color on the walls, to the color of your place setting, to the color of your food—all these can nurture balance and serenity within you. It's amazing how simply changing the wall color can affect your mood.
5. Fragrance—Throughout my home, I always have fragrant plants and flowers, as well as scented candles, as these restore balance and peace and promote relaxation. Your dining area and home should be a sanctuary and your meals a peaceful experience in order to nourish body and soul.

In her book, *Eating in the Light*, Doreen Virtue, PhD writes, "A major link between eating and one's spiritual path is to eat foods that nurture and support you. Take time to experiment with different foods so you can determine which ones truly work for you." I agree. Be patient with yourself. It took you years, maybe decades, to eat the way you're eating. Don't expect to change your entire diet overnight. Listen to Pythagorus, who said, "Choose what is best; habit will soon render it agreeable and easy."

It's very simple. By eating more fresh fruits and vegetables, with at least 50 percent of your diet consisting of wholesome living foods, and by practicing a few common-sense guidelines like drinking more water, eating more slowly, chewing your food well, and creating a peaceful environment in which to eat, you'll be feeling and showing the benefits in no time. Your friends will start asking what you're doing differently, because you exude energy and vitality, look and feel years younger, look at things with a more positive, graceful attitude, and live more serenely. You have brought a sacred balance into your body and life.

SIX OF MY FAVORITE COMPANIES AND HEALTHY LIVING PRODUCTS

Each year, I receive more than 2,000 letters asking about my favorite nutritional supplements and health products. Three of them have been part of my program for 40 years.

The first is the Penn Herb Company Ltd. In business since 1924, they offer America's most unique source for medicinal herbs and natural remedies. I learned about Penn Herb in the early 1970s from my grandmother, Fritize, who taught me how to take care of my body from head to toe, inside and out, using only natural remedies. As a teenager I had terrible allergies, along with a variety of other ailments, and she had me use some of the world-famous Olbas Remedies from Penn Herb Company. Everyone should keep the entire line of Olbas Remedies in their natural medicine chest: Olbas Inhaler, Olbas Sugar-Free Lozenges, Olbas Oil, Olbas Cough Syrup, Olbas Pastilles, Olbas Herbal Bath, Olbas Instant Herbal Tea, and Olbas Analgesic Salve. They help relieve aches and pains, enhance breathing passages, cool sore throats, and calm coughs. Olbas Oil, which I use many times weekly with clients or myself, originated in Basel, Switzerland over 100 years ago. This unique oil contains six essential oils: peppermint, eucalyptus, cajeput, wintergreen, juniper berry, and clove. Each of these oils has a unique value of its own. They are carefully extracted from traditional plants and blended by Swiss herbalists to make the formula truly unique.

Penn Herb Company offers more than 5,000 natural products, although the ones I purchase the most are the complete line of the Olbas Remedies and their Nature's Wonderland products. In my books and in radio and TV interviews, workshops, and health retreats worldwide, I am always extolling the virtues of this esteemed company and their complete product line. With the help of all their natural products, I have never taken medication in my life. My natural medicine cabinet is filled with remedies from Penn Herb Company. For a free sample of Olbas, visit *www.PennHerb.com*.

Second is one of my favorite supplements. The extract used in most garlic scientific studies, Kyolic Aged Garlic Extract, is revered worldwide. It has been proven effective in almost 700 studies—far more than all the other garlic products combined. That's because Aged Garlic Extract works for prevention and treatment of an amazing number of ailments—and it literally works wonders. I've perused most of the studies and have been so impressed that I've taken Kyolic for 40 years! One of the pluses of Kyolic is that you can remain "sociable" even while ingesting garlic— it's completely odorless.

Are you searching for a natural way to spark and strengthen your immune system? The medical community discovered Kyolic and the efficacy of its twelve- to fourteen-month aging process, which gives it the power to protect and enhance the health of our trillions of cells. Well-documented studies from major medical universities around the world have found Kyolic Aged Garlic Extract, an unheated, all-natural, health-promoting supplement, to be effective in its ability to resist and fight cancer, cardiovascular disease, other respiratory ailments and infections, and fatigue.

It also shows promise against homocysteine—a major risk factor in Alzheimer's disease and atherosclerosis.

In a recent one-year study conducted at UCLA Harbor School of Medicine, research leader Matthew J. Budoff, MD, became a believer in the efficacy of Kyolic. Kyolic Aged Garlic Formula 108 (B-12, B-6, Folic Acid, L-Arginine, and Kyolic) was proven more effective than the statin, aspirin, and placebos in all of the following categories: eight times more effective at inhibiting coronary calcification, four and a half times more effective in lowering homocysteine, two times more effective in increasing HDL levels, eighteen times more effective in preventing the oxidation of LDL, and three times more effective in lowering total cholesterol—all without negative side effects. And the patients took just four capsules per day of Kyolic Formula 108. The results speak for themselves. Dr. Budoff now says, "Take Aged Garlic Extract, it may save your life."

Kyolic comes in a variety of formulas, depending on your health concerns and goals, and each formula earns an A-plus in my book. For more detailed information on Kyolic Aged Garlic Extract, or for a free sample, please visit *www.kyolic.com*.

The third product that I highly recommend and wouldn't be without is Glutathione (GSH), the master antioxidant in the body. To stay healthy and prevent disease, it's the most important molecule, yet you've probably never heard of it. In my research on this remarkable antioxidant, I've found that it's one of the best secrets I know to slow down aging and prevent dementia, cancer, heart disease, and more, and it is also necessary to treat everything from autism to Alzheimer's disease. There are more than 79,000 medical articles about it—and chances are that your doctor doesn't know about the epidemic deficiency of this critical life-giving molecule.

While the body produces some glutathione, the bad news is that medications, stress, pollution, poor diet, toxins, trauma, aging, infections, and radiation all deplete your glutathione levels. This leaves you susceptible to unrestrained cell disintegration from oxidative stress, free radicals, infections, and cancer. As a result, your liver gets overloaded and damaged, making it unable to do its job of detoxification.

If you are over the age of twenty I recommend that you take a glutathione-accelerator.

In my private practice, I have seen it help improve mental function, increase energy, improve concentration, enhance exercise endurance, improve heart and lung function, and promote better sleep—just to name a few benefits. When optimal levels of GSH are available, a person often experiences renewed energy as well as radiant health.

Up until a few years ago, there was very little we could do to facilitate the body's innate ability to maintain optimal production of glutathione. The most efficient way to increase GSH levels was by intravenous injection, since supplemental forms of glutathione are virtually useless as they are degraded in the stomach environment. But thanks to over ten years of extensive research by Robert Keller, MD, we now have available a remarkable supplement, MaxGXL—the glutathione accelerator that has been scientifically proven to increase the body's ability to produce this master antioxidant at the cellular level by as much as 300 percent with three-month consecutive use.

For more information on MaxGXL, you can visit my website and click on *Maximize Health*. I encourage you to take it for three months and see for yourself how much better you will feel and look. To order a three-month supply, visit *www.4HealthBliss.com* or, to order wholesale, simply call (801)-316-6380 and tell them about my recommendation. MaxGXL has made a positive difference in my life; I know it will do the same for you, too.

My fourth nutritional supplement recommendation is Aphanizomnenon flos-aquae (AFA). For thousands of years, algae have been used worldwide as an excellent food source and potent medicine. For 25 years, the naturally occurring AFA growing in Oregon has been harvested and sold as a unique dietary supplement that's teeming with health-promoting compounds. "Although AFA grows in many other areas of the world," writes Christian Drapeau in his book, *Primordial Food Aphanizomenon flos-aquae: A Wild Blue-Green Alga with Unique Health Properties*, "the biomass that accumulates every year in Klamath Lake is unique in its abundance as well as its purity."

E3Live™ is 100 percent AFA. It's available in its complete fresh frozen liquid form. E3Live is collected only from the deepest, most primitive waters of Klamath Lake, Oregon, and harvested only at peak times of optimal growth, when the AFA is the heartiest4. For over 12 years, I've taken E3Live consistently, used it in my private practice, and highly recommend it to everyone. It provides more chlorophyll than wheatgrass; 60 percent high quality protein; all the B vitamins, including B-12; essential omega-3 and omega-6 fatty acids; and powerful digestive enzymes. It's also organic, kosher, vegan, raw, and versatile.

E3Live is an abundant source of phycocyanin. Similar to chlorophyll, phycocyanin protects your body against toxins found in food, air, and water. It also promotes healthy joint function and is an effective antioxidant. Similarly, E3Live is rich in PEA, a compound naturally produced by the brain that's released when we experience feelings of love, joy, and mental awareness. When taken orally, it is known to readily cross the blood-brain barrier and become immediately available to the brain. E3Live is the feel-good food—an excellent source of PEA.

In my work with clients, I've seen E3Live help in the following ways: promote natural weight loss; reverse premature aging; increase strength and endurance; improve memory and concentration; stabilize mood swings; normalize cholesterol levels; promote strong nails, smooth skin, and healthy hair; and provide deep sleep. Simply put: it gives you the full spectrum of over 64 perfectly balanced, naturally occurring vitamins, minerals, amino acids, and essential fatty acids. E3Live provides immediate 97 percent nutrient absorption, nourishing the body at the cellular level and helping to restore overall biological balance.

Commit to taking E3Live for 90 days and see how great you feel. For more information on this product and others, visit my website. To order, visit *www.E3Live.com.*

And finally, my fifth and sixth favorite products are front and center in my healthy kitchen. These are two angel gadgets or kitchen machines that I'd never be without. One is the Blendtec Total Blender and the other is the Ionizer Plus Water Electrolyzer. Both of these angel gadgets make it really easy to be radiantly healthy and forever younger. Rather than going into detail here, I encourage you to visit my website, *www.SusanSmithJones.com,* and click on "Favorite Products" to read more on why I highly recommend these products to everyone. I even give them away as gifts.

Eat to live, don't live to eat; many dishes, many diseases.
—BENJAMIN FRANKLIN

CHAPTER 8

Experience Ecstasy
I CHOOSE TO TURN MY DREAMS INTO REALITY

*Shake yourself awake. Let the winds of enthusiasm
sweep through you. Live today with gusto.*
—DALE CARNEGIE

*The way for you to be happy and successful, to get more of the things
you really want in life, is to get the combinations to the locks. Instead of
spinning the dials of life hoping for a lucky break, as if you were playing a
slot machine, you must instead study and emulate those who already have
done what you want to do and achieved the results you want to achieve.*
—BRIAN TRACY

People often say we create our own reality. In fact I've been suggesting it throughout this book. But what does that really mean? A few years ago I had an amazing experience that showed me.

I was accustomed to going to the beach for an invigorating swim a few times each week, very early, and this was a splendid morning just before sunrise. After some stretching exercises and a short run, I was ready for my swim. Because it was the end of summer, the water was still comfortably warm. But this morning there was something in the air that I couldn't quite identify. I felt it deep inside me—a shiver of anticipation, a faint knowing that today would be different, that this day would be one I would remember the rest of my life. I went out into the ocean, rode a few waves, and then swam past the swells.

I was aware of the peacefulness of the water. Sparkling and resplendent, it rejuvenated my body and soul with each stroke. A few minutes later some old friends joined me—a group of pelicans who seemed to enjoy escorting me. These marvels of nature have always enthralled me. They were gliding flawlessly a few feet above my head, their wingspans so large that they almost eclipsed the light, when suddenly they flew away. Surprised, I waved good-bye as I turned over to begin the backstroke. It was then I saw something that made my heart plummet.

A large, dark, frightening fin was heading straight for me. Shark! I looked toward the beach. No one was there. I had always taken for granted that I would stay calm in a life-threatening situation. But not this time! As the fin continued in my direction, I simply froze and treaded water. I was so terrified, I couldn't swim away or even cry out. And then it happened—a sight that will forever warm my heart and soul. The fin danced out of the water. It was a dolphin, and it was followed by a school of about two dozen more!

Less than two weeks before, I had watched a television documentary on dolphins. During my meditation that evening, I had visualized myself swimming and playing with a school of dolphins. I accepted and affirmed that that was my desire and reality. I then thanked God for this wonderful experience.

There in the ocean that morning, the dolphins stayed with me for a full half-hour, swimming, jumping out of the water, and jumping over me. I swam underwater with them, listening to their mellifluous sounds, touching their skin and feeling a connection and an exchange of love. For what seemed like hours, nothing else existed except my world of dolphins. I was oblivious to any thought of the past or future and lived right in the moment, rejoicing in the thrill of discovery.

Then, as quickly as they had arrived, the dolphins swam off, and I was left alone and immensely grateful. I swam back to shore, where by now a group of people had gathered, captivated by my dance with the dolphins. I answered many questions and tried to share what the experience had been like for me, but I found it very hard to put my feelings into words. Experiences that speak directly to the heart are often ineffable and difficult to express clearly through words.

The other people on the beach drifted away and I just sat there, enveloped in wonder at the experience of swimming with dolphins, and all I could do was cry—what had happened touched me so lovingly, so profoundly. What a beautiful lesson in living in the present and appreciating each moment. Because of that experience and so many others, I will never doubt the power of thought and belief to create any reality we choose.

PUTTING OUR THOUGHTS TO WORK

In the 1970s positive thinking became almost synonymous with success. In its early use in contexts such as Dale Carnegie's success courses, positive thinking meant using willpower and conscious, positive thoughts to achieve goals. Napoleon Hill's maxim for success, "What you can conceive and believe, you can achieve," was a popular positive thinking slogan. Never underestimate the Divine potential of positive thinking. Rightly employed, this power of the mind is a catalyst that makes possible a wondrous transformation in our lives. It was Ralph Waldo Emerson who said, "The good mind chooses what is positive, what is advancing—embraces the affirmative."

Positive thinking includes belief in our own self-worth and in the value of everyone else and every circumstance. Such positive belief leads to self-confidence, respect for others, and a lifestyle based on strong values. Sometimes we slip into the habit of negative thinking because we feel discouraged, depressed, lonely, isolated, or stressed. We all want fast and easy results. But life isn't like that. Life is meant to be a challenge, and one of its greatest lessons is that when our minds are full of fear, doubt, and clutter, good ideas can't get through. The best ideas and best decisions come when we're relaxed and open to impressions and responsive to them. In that state, we can find a way to link the present situation with wonderful opportunities to learn and grow.

Don't try to sit in a chair and think positively about something and expect it to happen. Keeping alive a goal or dream, or even hope, requires action. You have to make it happen—or at least help make it happen.

TAKE CHARGE OF YOUR MIND AND LIFE

You'll notice that successful people are very deliberate about choosing to be in charge of their lives. They don't get up in the morning and hope that they'll have a good day. High-achieving people take full control of their lives and, if they don't encounter the circumstances they want, they make them. Success and real fulfillment always begin with a dream. Successful people know nothing will happen unless they have the courage to start living their dream. This means taking risks, being vulnerable, making mistakes, and even failing. Life can't be lived on the sidelines if you want to be successful. There's enormous fun, as well as risk, in challenging yourself to something you've always wanted to do.

Too often we live in our comfort zone instead of taking risks. How often did your mom tell you "Take a risk today, sweetie!" when she sent you off to school? Probably never. Most of us are taught from a very early age to play small and play it safe rather than to play big and expand our horizons. Our comfort zone can remain tiny all our lives unless we subject it to some growing pains.

The way we live reflects our thoughts, dreams, expectations, beliefs, hopes, feelings of self-worth, and desires. We have free will to create our own happiness and our own heaven or hell. Here's a quick example of how we create our own reality: One of my clients, Kathleen, doesn't like where she lives but she can't afford to move. She resided in an old, noisy apartment building where her walls were in need of a fresh coat of paint, the windows hadn't been washed in years, and she didn't have any plants or other living things besides herself and her cat. It was no surprise to me that she was miserable, had a hard time sleeping, lacked energy, and felt depressed. She complained about her surroundings often in our counseling sessions, but failed to do anything about it—until I presented her with a challenge and assignment. I explained to her that if she would simply paint some of the walls a soothing color such as soft green or pale blue or teal, bring in some fresh flowers and plants and get a simple water fountain and perhaps a sound device (that plays the sounds of nature such a ocean waves, gentle rain, and singing birds, etc.) to help block out the noisy neighbors, she would be much happier in her environment, sleep better, and have a more positive attitude. And then I said that if she would do this in the next week, I would gift her with a dinner party and make all of the food for five of her favorite friends. Well, that put a smile on her face. In fact, she got so excited about these few changes—which cost less than $150.00—that she used a few days of vacation time at work to get the projects done within four days. During the dinner party, everyone loved her personal and physical changes, and we all could feel her energy shift. She had gone from feeling sad, depressed, and enervated to being happy, hopeful, and energetic.

What can you change in your immediate surroundings today, this week, this month that will also put a smile on your face and in your heart? Knowing this, you can consciously modify your inner states to create and live your highest potential and vision. You are not the victim of circumstances; you are the architect of your life. Your conscious thoughts create an unconscious image of your life, yourself, and your feelings, and that unconscious image reproduces itself perfectly in your real-life circumstances.

When life gets complicated and we find ourselves with negative thoughts and feelings, it's tempting to think that it's the complications, conditions, or people that upset us. But that's not the way it really works. It's only the way we think about the things that happen to us that cause our upsets. We can choose not to become upset. We really can. And as we change our thoughts and stop thinking of ourselves as victims, our lives shift and change in all kinds of positive ways.

HOW TO BREAK THE VICIOUS CYCLE OF NEGATIVE THINKING

Let's look at an all-too-common example of how the principle of choice works: weight control. Let's just assume that you've always had difficulty controlling your weight. You've tried all kinds of diets and they've never worked, so you have negative feelings about diets. You've tried to limit the amount of food you eat without much success, so you don't have much faith in your self-control. You get on the scale every morning and it reinforces your image of yourself as overweight. It really is a vicious cycle. In order to understand why you keep repeating the same patterns, you need to understand the way your mind works.

Brain researchers see the mind as composed of three primary parts: the conscious, the subconscious, and the super-conscious. As your window to the world, the conscious mind runs your daily waking activities, such as making decisions, relating to others, and doing your work. The subconscious mind, at the same time, carries memories of all your experiences. It is a storage-and-retrieval center for all the information your conscious mind sends it based on your daily experiences—essentially a computer that is fed the data of your every thought, feeling, and experience. The superconscious mind is your connection to the Divine. I talked about the superconscious in chapter 6 on meditation.

Relating this to the example of weight control, if you get up every morning and worry about what clothes will fit, if you dread getting on your scale, if you dislike being seen in public, if you think about going on a diet but doubt that it will work (they don't—I've written about that extensively in my books), you are programming your subconscious computer with negative thoughts. Your subconscious mind creates reality according to its programming. If you think of yourself as being fat, having little self-control, or being unable to change, you will see those beliefs reflected in your life—and you won't lose a pound.

The same is true for every other area of your life. Your subconscious beliefs and thoughts about yourself, your relationships with others, your money, your material possessions, your job, and so on, will be faithfully re-created in your life. You may be thinking, "No, that isn't true for me: I know that I really want to lose weight and tone up my body (or make more money, or have a really good relationship), but I am not experiencing it in my life." The answer lies in the vast difference between wanting something on the conscious level and wanting it on the subconscious level.

The conscious mind and the subconscious mind are often in conflict. Consciously you may want something, yet subconsciously you create mediocrity or failure. That's why positive thinking as it's commonly perceived doesn't work. As I lecture around the country and the world, I often hear statements such as, "I continually affirm, visualize, meditate, and believe in my highest good, but I rarely see results." It doesn't do much good to force yourself to think positive thoughts if your subconscious still harbors many negative beliefs. What you need to do is to reprogram your subconscious mind to break the vicious cycle of negative beliefs creating your negative reality. In order to do this, you must make some behavior changes on a conscious level that will contribute to new beliefs.

The birth of excellence begins with our awareness that our beliefs are a choice. We can choose beliefs that limit us, or we can choose beliefs that support us. The key is to choose beliefs that are conducive to success and to discard the ones that hold you back. Beliefs can turn on or shut off the flow of ideas. Our beliefs are what determine how much of our potential we'll be able to tap. Virgil, one of the greatest poets of ancient Rome, said, "They can because they think they can."

WHAT YOU THINK ABOUT, YOU BRING ABOUT

In the world of metaphysics, there is an unwritten law of correspondence that says, "As within, so without." The way I explain this in my workshops is that we are always attracting to ourselves the equivalency of what we think, how we feel, and what we believe. Ralph Waldo Emerson said that we become what we think about all day long. In other words, your outer world tends to be a reflection of your inner (subconscious) world—like a mirror. What you see in the world around you will be consistent over time with the world inside you.

Studies reveal that successful, happy people think about successful, happy things most of the time. By the same token, unsuccessful, unhappy people concentrate their thoughts on people they dislike, situations they are angry about, and events that they do not wish to take place in their lives. These data point directly to the law of concentration, which says, "Whatever you dwell upon grows in your reality." These ideas come from all of the great masters in life—from people like Buddha, Jesus, Socrates, Pythagoras, Thoreau,

Emerson, and Whitman. If you saw the DVD or read the book called *The Secret*, you are aware of these "laws of the universe" that have come down through the ages and, when implemented in our lives, will transform us if we embrace them.

These two laws in combination explain much of success and most of failure. Whatever we think about most of the time, we bring about in our lives.

So the starting point in making your dreams a reality is to discipline yourself to think and talk about only those things you want in your life, and to refuse to think and talk about anything other than what you want. These can be intangible as well as tangible things. Besides thinking and talking about the new job or material things you desire, talk and think about healthy things, such as being grateful. Try being loving instead of angry. Push aside all of that negativity—all of those fears, doubts, and self-sabotaging, limiting thoughts and visions—and you will discover that all manner of remarkable things happen in your life that bring you closer to your dreams.

It's equally important to feel the feeling of the dream fulfilled, of whatever it is you desire, whether it's being prosperous, fit, and healthy; being in a loving, supportive relationship; or being very successful at work. If you start acting a certain way, you eventually become that way. The key to the process is to capture the feeling, because when you do that you've captured the ability to internalize your idea, and then it's only a matter of time. Feeling refers to the intensity or amount of emotion that accompanies your mental pictures.

Emotion is central to all accomplishments. You might want to remember the following: T x F = R: Thought times Feeling equals Realization. The thought or picture multiplied by the feeling or emotion that accompanies it equals the speed at which it occurs in your reality. This is something I created over 30 years ago to help my clients remember how important are their thoughts and feelings when they desire to create miracles in their lives.

My extensive research, as well as my own experience, has taught me to appreciate the importance of feelings. I like to describe emotion as an electromagnetic force field so strong that it sends up a vibration and pulls like vibrations to itself. It is a magnet for similar energy.

After interviewing many highly intelligent, successful people with diverse backgrounds and vast experience, I came to the conclusion that what we think about, and how we feel about the things we think about, are the determining factors in the way our life works out.

If we are thinking positive thoughts but not getting positive results, most of the time it's because the emotional channels have not been opened. This can be done by practicing forgiveness toward ourselves and others and by passionately releasing fear, anger, guilt, and any other feelings that block the presence of Love inside us.

When we see our world only according to what surrounds us right now, we limit what we are going to have. Instead of thinking "I'll believe it when I see it," try thinking "I'll see it when I believe it." In order for this process to work, you must also get in the habit of saying what it is you desire. Be specific. Specifically plant in your mind that which you choose to bring into your life. You see, the creative principle works according to the seeds you plant. If you plant scarcity, disease, and disaster, you get back scarcity, disease, and disaster. If you plant Love, you get back Love. Say what you want, be specific, and act as if what you want is already true. That's key.

Any feelings we want we can have, if we think intensely enough. Try it. It's remarkable, and it's true. We can even feel cool when it's hot or friendly when we'd rather be alone if we use our minds to paint the picture vividly enough. It's this powerful force of feeling, drawn into the subconscious mind, which acts as a generator to create what we desire.

POSITIVE ACTIONS BRING POSITIVE RESULTS

Here are some positive actions you can take to change your circumstances.

- If you feel that your beliefs about money are creating negative results in your life, examine the behaviors that support those negative beliefs. Maybe you are frugal in your grocery shopping, conscious of buying the cheapest brands and skipping the luxuries. Although frugality might be wise in light of your current financial situation, you should be aware that it also tends to reinforce your belief that you have very little money. One way to attack this belief is to substitute a new behavior for the old one. For example, the next time you're in a grocery store, allow yourself to indulge in a little luxury. While you're doing it, imagine that this capacity to indulge a little is your present reality, and feel it.
- If your problem is loneliness, make it a point to smile at one stranger every day, just as if you had plenty of friends and an abundance of Love to share.
- If you are heavier than you want to be, buy yourself something appealing that you would normally have denied yourself because of your present appearance.

SELF-ESTEEM

It's important to understand that living your vision and creating what your heart desires is related to how you feel about yourself. If you feel unworthy, it will be almost impossible for abundance to flow into your life. If you feel that you are important enough to ask and Divine enough to receive, receiving will be your reward. "Think of how a tree unfolds to all of its magnificent potential, always reaching for the sunshine and growing and flourishing," writes Wayne Dyer in

Change Your Thoughts—Change Your Life. "Would you ever suggest to a tree, 'You should be ashamed of yourself for having that disgusting moss on your bark and for letting your limbs grow crooked?' Of course not. A tree allows the Life Force to work through it. You have the power within your thoughts to be as natural as the tree." He reminds us that all we need to do is to be ourselves.

WHAT YOU GIVE AWAY, YOU GET BACK MULTIPLIED

Another important aspect of changing your subconscious energy involves the law of circulation, which states that what you give away, you get—multiplied. You must first give away the very thing you desire. If you desire increased prosperity in your life, for instance, don't hoard it, because that would be manifesting a fear that there might not be enough. Share what you have with others and feel how the world begins to open to you as well.

Once you decide what you want, begin tithing. Tithing traditionally means to give a tenth of your income to your church, but tithing doesn't necessarily have to go to a church—and it doesn't have to be ten percent. Tithe gifts can be in monetary form or a giving of yourself in time and/or deposits of Love. I tithe money to those who feed my soul and nourish my spirituality and who are making a positive difference on this planet, whether they are individuals or organizations. I also give money and time to people less fortunate than I. Remember, though, it's futile to say, "Yes, when such-and-such money comes in, I will give a tenth of it as a tithe." You have to start helping those in need before that, acting in the spirit of "give that you may receive."

One day, after writing my prosperity affirmations and goals on cards, I went to the grocery store. While waiting in the checkout line, I suddenly called out to the harried mother in front of me, "I'll pay for those." Needless to say, she was astonished! Quite honestly, so was I; the words seemed to have just popped out of my mouth. After some hesitancy on her part and some impressive cajolery on mine, she let me pay her bill. The pleasure I received made me feel rich inside. Later that same day, I ran into a person whom I had counseled several months before. At that time she had been unable to pay, and I had written the sessions off as a good learning experience. This day, seemingly out of the blue, she wrote me a check for twice the amount she owed me, saying that my guidance had a profound, positive effect on her life. I shouldn't have been surprised, because I had "acted as if."

To "act as if" takes courage and trust. It's hard to start giving when you don't think you have enough, unless you act as if. Go out into the world as if you had the courage, and you'll find that the courage you wanted is already there. Do the thing, and the power is yours. Yes, it begins with a risk, but if you don't risk, you don't receive. That's how you generate power.

Your subconscious mind is extraordinarily powerful, but it is a servant, not a master. It coordinates every aspect of your thoughts, feelings, behaviors, words, actions, and emotions to fit a pattern consistent with your dominant mental pictures. It guides you to engage in the behaviors that will move you ever closer to achieving the goals you visualize and feel most of the time. If you visualize something that you fear, your subconscious mind will accept that as a command, too. It will then use its marvelous powers to bring your fears, instead of your dreams and aspirations, into reality.

Many people feel that their deepest beliefs and motivations are forever a mystery to them. They feel they don't understand the real reasons behind their actions, and as a result they feel powerless to change their actions. They have it backwards: we all have the ability to recognize our beliefs through our actions, and to change them by changing our actions. Although beliefs may seem mysterious and complicated on a conscious level, on a subconscious level they are usually simple. Our beliefs about ourselves are based entirely on our past experiences. All of our experiences program our subconscious, and the result is what we are today.

That is not to say that all you will ever be is the sum of your experiences. Maybe you've noticed at some time or other that your life experiences are all very similar—it's just the people involved who keep changing. You can change that pattern by choosing to feed different programming into your subconscious computer.

CHOOSE YOUR THOUGHTS AND WORDS WISELY

Two very effective ways to reprogram your subconscious mind are creative visualizations and affirmations. The idea is to alter your state of consciousness in such a way that you can temporarily set aside the conscious mind and concentrate specifically on the subconscious. According to brain researchers, suggestions given to your subconscious while in this altered state, whether they are images or affirmations, will be at least twenty times as effective as suggestions given in a normal state of consciousness. One of the best ways to alter or slow down your state of consciousness or brain wave activity is through relaxed deep breathing.

It's very helpful to feed your mind a clear mental picture of your desired goals for the coming day, the coming week, and the coming months just before going to sleep at night. I do this every night for about ten minutes. As you drop off to sleep, your brain wave activity naturally slows down and your subconscious mind is the most receptive to the input of new commands. Since your mental pictures are a command, take those last few minutes before you fall asleep to daydream and fantasize about exactly the person you want to be and the life you want to have. Your subconscious mind will then take the pictures down into its laboratory and work on them all night long. What often happens is that you wake up in the morning with ideas and insights that will help make those things you visualized a part of your life.

Most people have only vague, fuzzy pictures of what they want. They say they want to be rich or healthy or happy. But when you ask them exactly what that means to them, they don't really know. In his book *Maximum Achievement*, Brian Tracy, renowned for his work on the powers of the mind and visualization, emphasizes the importance of vividness in mental pictures. The more vividly you can see something that you want in your mind's eye, he says, the more rapidly it will materialize in your reality.

Vividness requires precision and clarity of detail in your mental pictures. Spend some time examining your desired goals, drawing pictures of them either actually or mentally, or writing out clear descriptions of what your wishes would look like when they came true. Complex pictures will be accepted by your subconscious as a command, and your subconscious mind will go immediately to work to coordinate all your other resources, internal and external, to bring those goals into your life.

Be precise. Be absolutely definite. Know what you want, visualize what you want, and say what you want. It will not do to say you want a lot of money or that you want a new car or a house. You must state exactly what it is that you want and hold that picture steadily before you, so strongly that you can feel the wish fulfilled.

If you want money (though if you are wise, you will not bother much about money—no one has ever taken a single coin into the next world), state definitely how much you want. It must be a definite sum. If prosperity is your goal, make part of your visualization definite plans for the good you will do with the prosperity you create.

Your visualizations can be turned into affirmations by making them real and vivid in your mind. Write down your major goals in the present tense on three-by-five cards, one to a card, and review them on a regular basis. Read the goal—for example, "I have an hour each day for myself"—then close your eyes, breathe deeply, relax for a few seconds, and imagine what it would be like if you did indeed have that hour. Visualize some of the specific ways your life would change. Feel the feeling of calm and groundedness that comes with that extra time. Then open your eyes, smile, and go about your business, knowing in your mind's eye that you have already succeeded in achieving your goal.

A few years ago, one of my goals and dreams was to have a home-away-from-home, somewhere out in a natural setting where I could go to write and have some quiet and solitude. Although I wasn't sure where I wanted this home to be, I was very clear on some of my specific requirements: I wanted it to be a long way from a large city and crowds of people, and surrounded by trees and nature's sounds. The home itself needed to be made of wood and windows, have a spectacular view, and lend itself to my healthy lifestyle—sun, fresh air, organic garden, and space to work out. So for a few months I visualized this home. I wrote my vision down on three-by-five index cards and gave thanks that it was already a reality.

About six months later, I was invited to give a seven-day workshop in a town on the coast of Oregon. I had been there before, speaking at Unity and other churches and at the local hospital. I had always thought it was a beautiful area but had never considered buying a home there. One evening I had a break during my workshop and was invited to visit some friends who lived on top of a forested hill overlooking the Pacific. During our conversation in their home, they mentioned that the house next door was for sale. I answered casually and didn't give the information any more thought until later: in the middle of the night I was hit by a cosmic two-by-four and immediately realized I was supposed to buy that house next door to my friends. The realization seemed absurd, because I hadn't even looked at the inside of the house. I simply knew it was meant to be mine, and that it would be the perfect place for personal retreats and writing.

The next morning I called my friends. They were delighted with my decision, even though they thought I was a little crazy! I called the realtor, and learned that the house was already in escrow, about to close. He would be happy to show me other homes, he said, but this one was no longer available. I told him, "You don't seem to understand. That's my home and I'm not interested in looking at any others." I left my telephone number and asked him to call me when the house was available. You can guess how the story turned out: it did become available, I made an offer, and it became my retreat home.

It certainly didn't come without roadblocks—the path of least resistance isn't always the best one. The whole process of creating my home presented me with one challenge after another and taught me numerous lessons as well, such as the importance of belief and faith and not judging by appearances; such as being thankful for everything seen and unseen, and beholding the Divine in everyone and everything. By the way, my home-away-from-home is on top of a hill, surrounded by trees, overlooking the bay, has lots of light, and is filled with angels, just as I visualized it. I had never thought about that specific location, but I know, now that I have it, that it's the perfect place for me and was made possible because of my focused desire for it.

TAKE A WORD INVENTORY

Like most of us, from time to time I get into bad habits with words. Not too long ago, I was driving with my close friend, Reverend John Strickland. The day was hot and the traffic was heavy. A rude, reckless driver cut me off. I said in a loud voice, "I hate it when someone does that to me!" John looked very startled. He said, "Don't use the 'H' word. That's a terrible thing to put into your consciousness. Try instead, 'I prefer drivers not to cut me off in traffic,' and then silently bless the driver."

I was in no mood to listen to a lecture. I felt like saying to him, "I hate it when somebody lectures me!" But I didn't do that, because he was absolutely correct. Have you ever said, "That burns me up," "They're driving me crazy," or "This is backbreaking work"? These seemingly harmless expressions program garbage into your subconscious mind. The subconscious does not know that you don't really mean it. It plants those ideas in your experience storage and plays them out into your life as if you really meant what you said. Just as an injurious diet weakens the body, leading inevitably to disease, a regimen of negative thoughts and words debilitates the mind and soul, fostering unhappiness and an unfulfilled life.

Take an inventory of everything you say during the course of the day. Be aware of the words you use. Speak only those words that are positive, loving, and uplifting, and that represent what you want for yourself.

I've learned to pay attention to what I say (most of the time) and to interrupt negative expressions. When I find myself straying toward negativity, I usually say or think "cancel" or "erase" and then change the words. I have also imagined in my mind's eye a large screen on which I write any negative expressions I've used and then draw an X through them. I have done this on paper, too, and then burned the paper. Use any method that is effective for you.

It can be a real challenge to find positive ways to say exactly what you mean. But it certainly can be done. For instance, notice how often you say "I'm sorry" and try "I apologize" instead. After all, that is what you mean. Change "I'm afraid you have the wrong number" to "You have the wrong number." For "I hate it when my boss is in a bad mood," try "I prefer a cheerful workplace." As you find more ways to speak more accurately, you stop feeding your subconscious mind misinformation about yourself.

You are as good as your word. In my opinion, when it comes to keeping your word, there is no such thing as a small situation. Perhaps it's no big deal to say we're going to call someone and then not do it, but it can be very important to the other person. It's very important to me that my friends and business associates be accountable—that their words count. When I learn that someone doesn't follow through on what they say they're going to do, and it's apparent that this is a pattern, I choose not to spend time with that person. To me, a verbal agreement is as serious and binding as a written one. In fact I have verbal agreements, as opposed to written ones, with most of the companies for which I do consulting. People know my word is good and they can count on me.

I'm very inspired by people who make their word count. My mom, June, was always a shining example for me of the importance of keeping your word. Every time she made a promise, no matter how small or seemingly insignificant, she kept her word. If she made plans with someone and then was offered the opportunity to do something more exciting or interesting, she never hesitated one second before she would say, "Thank you, I'd love to do it, but I already have a commitment." June's behavior invariably brought two reactions, both positive. The first friend was pleased because she and June did whatever they were going to do, and the second friend was impressed with her integrity. June was not only well-liked, she was also very successful. She was as good as her word. To me, there can be no higher praise than that.

Make your word count. It's a gift you give to your family, friends, business associates, community, and the world.

In a study conducted at Sussex University, subjects viewed a selection of television news broadcasts. The topics were positive, negative, or neutral. Not surprisingly, negative news broadcasts left the subjects in a bad mood and made most of them edgy. We always have a choice about what we look at and to what we give our attention. So reinforce positive thoughts, words, and actions by what you watch, and avoid putting your attention on negativity. Thoughts embroiled in negativity tarnish your perception of the beauties and miracles of life. Fill not only your conversation but your consciousness with positive things. Surmount all life's challenges by following your heart and letting the Divine wisdom within you guide you to the realization of your dreams.

PATIENT PERSISTENCE IN THE GOOD

There's an unfathomable, yet recognizable, Divine Order to this universe. It's ever-present and always working in alignment with what we need for our highest good and spiritual unfolding and growth. I've learned not to analyze or question it anymore. It asks only for our trust, faith, and courage.

You are exactly where you need to be in life. At any moment you can choose to experience something else, simply by taking responsibility and consciously choosing to think differently. In the fantastic words of *Zorba the Greek* writer Nikos Kanzantzakis, "You have your paintbrush and colors. Paint paradise, and in you go."

When we narrow things down to the essentials, we discover what we most value.
—ALEXANDRA STODDARD

Hope is one of the best ways to shed light on the process of unfolding miracles—and it's part of the ongoing miracle itself.
—THOMAS KINKADE

CHAPTER 9

Seek Opportunities for Service and Stillness

I CHOOSE A LIFE OF TRUE QUALITY

To affect the quality of the day, that is the highest of arts.
—HENRY DAVID THOREAU

Learn to get in touch with the silence within yourself and know that everything in this life has a purpose.
—ELISABETH KÜBLER-ROSS

SERENITY

When you come from an empowered presence and feel confidence aplenty because you see your life changing for the better before your eyes, as you learned how to do in the previous chapter, you open your life to abundant joy. Your self-esteem soars, you smile more, and you feel more connected to life and miracles all around you just waiting for your acknowledgment. This is what living fully is all about: Creating our very best lives and living with a peaceful serenity because we know that we are not mere victims of circumstance; we are the architects of our lives, the master of our ship, the producer, director, and actor of our play.

I don't know about you, but I want to create a romantic, comedy adventure rather than a depressing, tragic drama. I want a life of quality, a life of joy. So, what pursuits toward this end have we not yet covered, what choices have we not considered? I can think of only two: serenity and service.

Thomas Alva Edison, the great inventor, was a true master of the art of serenity. When his factory burned down, he did not spend time bemoaning his fate. The newspaper reporters who went to interview him immediately following the disaster found him calmly at work on plans for a new building.

Another master of this art was Ralph Waldo Emerson. As his house burned and his library of precious books went up in flames, writer Louisa May Alcott tried to console him. The philosopher said to her, "Yes, yes, Louisa, they're all gone, but let's enjoy the blaze now."

According to Webster's dictionary, serenity is "the quality or state of being serene"—calm, tranquil, untroubled, steady, quiet. Not surprisingly, in order to master the art of serenity, we need also to master the art of being alone.

SILENCE

There's an old saying that God gave us two ears and one mouth so we might hear more and talk less. How well we use our ears plays an important part in determining what we learn as we go through life. I find that I am more peaceful and more serene when I listen more and talk less.

Although it's almost impossible to find absolute silence in the outer world, we can always find silence inside. Mystics, saints, and spiritual leaders of the past and present have all advocated periods of silence for spiritual growth and as a practical way to find balance and be made whole again. Through the regular practice of silence they have all been able to achieve solitude, even when they were in the presence of others.

It's hard to experience silence when we are constantly bombarded with the noises that seem to be part of living in our technological society. They aren't necessarily loud noises, but they are pervasive. Just try and seek some quiet time to yourself and you'll become more sensitive to subtle sounds such as the refrigerator motor, air conditioner, heater, washer and dryer, distant din of traffic, or nearby dripping faucet.

When I'm conducting a workshop in a natural setting, as I mentioned in a previous chapter, I often ask the participants to go outside for fifteen minutes and amble around the grounds alone in silence. I have them experience and practice being totally involved and absorbed in what they see, smell, feel, touch, or hear. I want them to let nature's beauty into their awareness through all their senses. No matter what part of the world we are in, participants come to me afterwards and say that this was their first experience of being truly alone and finding peace in their own company.

What I have discovered in taking this kind of walk is that I feel a subtle, gentle communion with nature. My entire being is rejuvenated as I seem to communicate with the flowers, trees, birds, clouds, butterflies, and even insects. I am more fully aware of my environment, sensitive to nature, and at one with all life. It is as if I have built a garden of the soul.

I devote a few hours a week to private counseling, and sessions with my clients might begin with an invigorating, conversation-free hike in the beautiful Santa Monica Mountains. I find this to be a wonderful way to let go and surrender to the spirit of life. Listening to the silence and sounds of nature is a great way to feel serene and in touch with our feelings, which makes it easier for us to express ourselves when we settle down to talk. By the time the session is over, we both feel rejuvenated physically, mentally, and spiritually.

Several years ago, I spent time in a monastery in which disciplined silence was required 24 hours a day. At first it was difficult. I was seeing, experiencing, and feeling so much that I wanted to share with others. Then, slowly and subtly, I discovered that the silence was overwhelmingly blissful. It was as though a gentle wave of peace swept over me. There was nothing but silence all around me, through me, and everywhere—expanding and spreading out to fill all creation. Things that touch the heart are often difficult to put into words, and this was one of those experiences. I just knew that I loved the silence, reveled in it, and wanted to have it with me always.

Ever since that experience, I have carried this silence with me. Even in conversation, I am aware of the quietness beneath the sounds of people's voices. Although I sometimes lose the awareness of it, I can recall it and let it once again be a source of great peace and joy, like the awareness of a close, loving friend. Remembering my time at the monastery, I now make sure I have regular periods of solitude and silence.

I recognize that I choose more solitude than most. Not only do I meditate at least twice a day but I also give myself several hours once a week, one weekend a month, and a few days with each change of season simply to be alone and embrace silence. In fact, as I write this chapter I am celebrating a new glorious season in Oregon, away from most of the activity of my usual world. This regular supplement of solitude and silence greatly enhances every area of my life. It nourishes my soul.

Silence and meditation are the best way I know to stay balanced. Constant activity and noise enervate the body and leave us feeling drained mentally, emotionally, and physically. Quality time alone is renewing. I enjoy exercising alone at dawn. I feel great not only because I am alone but also because I'm working out and finding pleasure in my own company. There is a sense of serenity in any solo activity—working or enjoying a bit of relaxation—that makes me feel complete, whole, and self-sufficient.

"Silence will help you see clearly exactly what is out of balance in your life," says Barbara De Angelis, PhD in her book *Real*

Moments. "It creates an opening through which you can receive truth, perspective, strength, healing, revelation."

Lying or withholding your true feelings darkens your soul, and deceit leads to unhappiness for everyone involved. Letting your feelings out is an expression of self-esteem; covering them up can be genuinely harmful to your health. In silence we can be honest with ourselves, and if we learn to tell the truth to ourselves, we can be honest with others. Nothing is more essential than honesty for your balance and serenity.

In silence, deep within our hearts, each of us knows the truth. If you persist in listening, you will learn to recognize and be led by the "still, small voice" within. However, finding this stillness doesn't happen overnight. "Through your persistent prayers for guidance and your calm receptivity," says Yogananda, "an inner sense will prompt you as to the best way to proceed. When that happens, go forward with full faith; but all the while remain flexible."

SOLITUDE

Another path to serenity is solitude. Every one of us needs time to discover the peace of our own company. While few of us would choose lifelong solitude, we can all benefit from some time to ourselves. We may differ from those around us in the extent, frequency, and urgency of our need for solitude, as well as in the way we spend our personal time. We may have trouble carving out periods of privacy, or even feel guilty about claiming them, but when we're deprived of them for too long, we experience distress and imbalance.

Some people are fearful of being alone, but remember, there is a huge difference between solitude and loneliness. These are the two sides of aloneness. Loneliness expresses the pain of being alone; solitude expresses the joy of being alone. Loneliness is usually not of our choosing, but solitude is.

Ah, solitude! Even the word evokes peace within me, perhaps because it's such a vital part of my life. Thoreau, one of my favorite mentors and inspirations, knew the joy of solitude:

> "It is a great relief when for a few moments in the day we can retire to our chamber to be completely true to ourselves. It leavens the rest of our hours." (Journal, March 20, 1841)

> "I have a great deal of company in my house; especially in the morning, when nobody calls." (Walden Pond)

> "I love to be alone. I never found a companion so companionable as solitude." (Walden Pond)

Sometimes finding time to be alone is a difficult thing. One of my friends has three children and rarely has time to herself. She works as well, and often finds herself rushing among the children's dance lessons, doctor appointments, grocery shopping, and different household errands. When she told me how she spends her days, I became exhausted just listening. I suggested she give herself permission to call some time her own. Now, after she drops off a child at dance class, she either pulls out a favorite book and reads in her car or spends time in meditation or just sitting in the park down the block from the dance studio. There are no phones, no people, and no distractions. She has created a salutary hour of quiet and serenity to do or think as she pleases.

In *Man's Eternal Quest*, Paramahansa Yogananda writes, "Be alone within. . . ." Enjoy solitude; but when you want to mix with others, do so with all your love and friendship, so that those persons cannot forget you, but remember always that they met someone who inspired them and turned their minds toward God."

Thoreau wrote something very similar in his Journal: "You think that I am impoverishing myself by withdrawing from men,

but in my solitude I have woven for myself a silken web or chrysa-
lis, and, nymph-like, shall ere long burst forth a more perfect crea-
ture, fitted for a higher society."

CARVING OUT TIME FOR SILENCE AND SOLITUDE

For some, solitary exercise may be all that is needed to stay balanced throughout the day. Others will want to spend several minutes alone one or more times a day in some form of meditation.
This spiritual exercise allows life's experiences to touch us more
gently. Still others might want to look into longer silent retreats,
to go more deeply into their own consciousness and clear all channels. Whether for short or extended periods of time, retreating
from the outside world can enhance and enrich all areas of our
lives.

If the issue is finding time, you must choose to make time.
Make privacy a priority in your life. Privacy is a universal need.
There will always be others who want some of your time. In order
to assure quiet time for yourself, reserve a regular period in your
daily schedule when your family and friends know that, barring
emergencies, you expect to be left alone. It is much easier when
you explain your needs clearly and specifically to others.

I believe that all the other good things we endeavor to provide
for ourselves—sound nutrition, daily exercise, nutritional supplements and health products, material plenty—are of limited value
unless we learn to live in harmony with ourselves, which means
knowing ourselves and finding peace in our own company. You'll
find that a greater peace is a natural consequence of spending
more time by yourself, especially once you realize that you are
never really alone and that you can live much more fully by focusing on inner guidance. Too often we look outside ourselves to find
our worth, forgetting that nothing will ever be enough until we

are enough. When we recognize that we are enough all by ourselves, everything else will be enough. It all starts on the inside.

When was the last time you were alone—I mean really alone—

and in silence, without radio, video, or tapes, listening to the

silence of your heart, being at peace with your own company?

Here are some simple ways to create and experience more silence
in your life:

- Drive with your radio turned off. Cars can be mobile awareness centers. Consider them "sacred spaces."
- Don't turn on your TV if you're not really watching. Background noise keeps your mind restless and open to unwant-
ed influences.
- Keep your telephone from becoming a disruptive force.
Turn the ringer off, and if you still have an answering machine turn the volume down a few days each week. If it's
workable, gather your messages at the end of the day and
return the calls in one sitting.
- Exercise without music or headphones. If you are outdoors,
listen to nature and move to the rhythm of your thoughts.
- Sit in silence by firelight or candlelight. "Watch the flames.
Listen to logs crackle, or watch the wax drip down the side
of the candle," says De Angelis. "Imagine the light illuminating all of the dark or hidden places inside of you. En-
joythe simplicity of the moment."
- Let nature nourish your soul. Sit quietly in a park or garden, or anywhere you can see water or hills or a tree. Listen to the whispering communication of plants, the rushing sounds of the birds' wings, or the breeze murmuring
through the leaves, and see the way the light reflects all the
colors of creation. Feel gratitude for all the beauty you see
around you.

- If you don't live near or have access to any natural environment, put on a nature tape and spend quality time in silence, listening to the marvelous sounds of the Earth. I keep many nature tapes and CDs on hand with sounds of birds, brooks, rain on trees, ocean waves, etc.
- Take a bubble bath with soothing essential oils.

SIMPLIFY, SIMPLIFY!

A natural outgrowth of the practices of solitude and silence is the desire to slow down and forego the hurry habit. It's an American sickness we've all seen growing over the past years: the "hurry" sickness, the "busyness" sickness. We see it everywhere—instant breakfasts, fast foods, in- and-out dry cleaners, one-minute managers, and 12-minute fitness programs. I wouldn't be surprised to see a new book about 30-second sex!

To let go of the busyness of life we must simplify our lives as much as possible. Simplify! It's a wonderful word, one that represents a powerful process. I have discovered great joy in simplifying all areas of my life: my thoughts, what I say, the ways I choose to spend my time, how I arrange my closets, cupboards, and garage—even my wishes and desires. I've became so good at simplifying, in fact, that my family and friends ask me to assist them with their process of simplification. What a delight to see lives transformed for the better, just by being pared down. My joy in seeing beauty and order around me has snowballed into another occupation, a business I call "Simply Organized," which involves working with clients to organize their homes and lives.

To simplify is so freeing, and it feels so good. It's hard to appreciate any one thing fully when too many are crammed together. This can be true of foods on the table, clothes in the closet, or pictures on the walls. You may have a fantastic collection of art objects in your home, but if they are crowded and cluttered, appreciating each piece is difficult.

Often we live so hurriedly that we don't pay attention to what's really important. Our lives are cluttered with things we don't need. When life gets too complicated and out of balance, we become less sensitive to our own needs and the needs of our family and friends. When we consciously choose to simplify, life seems to slow down, and we are better able to live in the present moment with an open awareness of our inner guidance and divinity.

Clean a closet, a cupboard, your garage.

What can you do to simplify your life right now, today? One surprisingly effective place to start is by cleaning out and simplifying one of your closets, some cupboards, or your garage. Spend 15 minutes each day, and keep it up until you have jettisoned everything you don't really want. Before you know it, your entire home will be transformed. As a result of this disciplined exercise, you will find yourself easily and naturally beginning to simplify other areas of your life—how you spend your time, what you think, and what you say. Simplifying the externals of life is not only freeing and refreshing, it also supports you in feeling more serene and peaceful and in seeing your life from a higher perspective. This technique works because outside and inside always reflect each other: change one and you influence the other.

Living fully and simply go hand in hand

In his book *Voluntary Simplicity*, Duane Elgin writes poignantly about the spiritual dimensions of simplicity:

To live with simplicity is to unburden our lives—to live a more direct, unpretentious, and unencumbered relationship with all aspects of our lives; consuming, working, learning, relating, and so on. Simplicity of living means meeting life face to face, confronting life clearly without unnecessary distractions, without trying to soften the enormity of our existence or masking the deeper manifestations of life with pretensions, distractions, and unnecessary accumulation. It means being direct and honest in relationships of all kinds. It means taking life as it is —straight and unadulterated.

Letting go of clutter, doing without pretensions, encumbrances, and superfluity is what living fully and joyfully is all about. Perhaps we can head in that direction by trying to be simpler and more selfless. The venerable Lao-Tzu said: "Manifest plainness, embrace simplicity, reduce selfishness, have few desires."

At one time in my life, I found great pleasure in collecting material things. My income was generous and I delighted in buying lots of clothes, appliances, gadgets, works of art, and cars, until it reached a point where I was seeking fulfillment from what I collected rather than from the Divinity within. In pursuit of material goals, I began to lose sight of the spiritual goals through which we achieve all fulfillment, happiness, and peace. I was looking outward to my collection of stuff rather than within, to my true nature, for worth as a human being.

Fortunately I discovered that what the world holds for me is not as important as what I bring to the world. When I realized that, it became clear to me that I wanted to simplify every aspect of my life. I have found that I can live simply and still live well. I buy clothes and other items these days, but more often I'm giving things away and finding ways to make my life less cluttered and complicated.

How can you simplify your life in order to fulfill your purpose more easily and gracefully? There isn't one answer for everybody. We can assist one another on our journey through this miracle called life, but no one can live your life for you. In the end, it all comes down to choice. Once you become aware that you are choosing everything, you can take over your own life and live it the way your Higher Self knows how to live it. You can choose to let go of clutter and complexity in favor of serenity, peace, and happiness—a more spiritual life.

TO FIND HAPPINESS, SERVE

The great gift that comes from simplifying is the gift of time. You have more time to slow down and focus on what's really important, like being of service and letting your inner guidance direct your thoughts, words, and actions. It's a relatively easy path for people who are lucky enough to be born with visions of peace and service: I remember that even when I was a child I wanted to speak to people about being happy and peaceful. I used to dream about visiting leaders of different countries all around the world and helping them resolve their conflicts. I believed in peace from the beginning, and I knew I wanted to be active and involved with health and fitness. I got in touch with those early visions when I grew up and made conscious, faith-filled choices based on them.

But anyone can cultivate the desire to serve. I believe that service is essential to a happy, spiritually guided life—and that service can also be the key to spiritualizing business. Yogananda said, "Instead of making money and greater profits your goal in business, make service your goal, and you will see the entire plan of your life change." That doesn't mean that we shouldn't enjoy a legitimate profit. It just means that if service, not money, is our goal, then profit follows automatically. Profit is the natural result of service. As the best entrepreneurs know, values can be profitable.

Whether or not we belong to a church or service organization or have a job that provides meaningful service opportunities, not one day goes by without some chance for us to serve another human being by making deposits of unconditional Love. Service isn't measured by specific deeds; the important thing is a loving, giving attitude. Someone once said, "Service is the rent we pay for the privilege of living on this earth." And there are so many ways to serve.

The greatest possible personal security comes from service, from helping other people in a meaningful way. One important source can be your daily work and seeing yourself in a contributing and creative mode, really making a difference. Another source is anonymous service that no one knows about and no one necessarily ever will. That's not your concern. Your only concern is blessing the lives of other people.

It is essential on any spiritual journey to be sure that your path is connected with your deepest Love. In *The Teachings of Don Juan*, Carlos Castañeda is told, "Look at every path closely and deliberately. Try it as many times as you think necessary. Then ask yourself and yourself alone one question. This question is one that only a very old man asks. My benefactor told me about it once when I was young and my blood was too vigorous for me to understand it. Now I do understand it. I will tell you what it is: Does the path have a heart? If it does, the path is good. If it doesn't, it is of no use." Serving others is one way to be sure that you are following a "path with heart."

Each day we can find ways to do some good. We can give to a worthy cause or help some individual with our time and loving care. Sometimes all a person needs is some understanding, attention, or compassion. See God in everyone, no matter how erring the person may be. One of my favorite affirmations is: "I behold the Divine in everyone and everything."

It is easier to see the Divine in other people if we've learned to see it in ourselves through solitude, silence, giving, and the unshakable serenity that comes from within. So begin today. Take an inventory of your life and the words, thoughts, actions, activities, and surroundings that fill your days. Ask yourself these questions:

1. What time can I carve out for quality solitude—daily, weekly, monthly, yearly?
2. What changes can I make in my home and office to eliminate clutter and beautify my surroundings?
3. When I have the choice of speaking or remaining silent, which will enhance the harmony of the situation?
4. In what ways can I delegate responsibilities or activities and allow others to serve me?
5. Whose life can I enrich in some fashion today, either with or without their awareness?
6. How can I deepen my relationship with Spirit today?

Out of clutter, find simplicity.
—ALBERT EINSTEIN

When we are authentic, when we keep our spaces simple, simply beautiful living takes place.
—ALEXANDRA STODDARD

The holiest of all holidays are those
Kept by ourselves in silence and apart,
The secret anniversaries of the heart . . .
—HENRY WADSWORTH LONGFELLOW

CHAPTER 10

Savor Balance in All Things
I CHOOSE THE SUREST PATH TO JOY

*It's terribly amusing how many different climates of feeling
one can go through in a day.*
—ANNE MORROW LINDBERGH

*God answers sharp and sudden on some prayers,
And thrusts the thing we have prayed for in our face,
A gauntlet with a gift in "it."*
—ELIZABETH BARRETT BROWNING

The idea that we have control over our wellness and that we can choose to be healthy and functioning at our best is far from new. What is new is this idea's growing popularity in the world of science and medicine. Immunologists, psychiatrists, endocrinologists, neuroscientists, microbiologists, and psychologists from around the world—professionals who rarely step outside their own fields—are combining their expertise in a new field called psychoneuroimmunology. This new science deals with the mind's effect on the body's incredibly complex network of organs, nerves, vessels, and white blood cells. Furthermore, research shows that the immune system, brain, and other vital body systems communicate, connect with, and influence one another.

Experts today are telling us that in almost every area, stress interferes with the body's ability to resist disease and heal itself. If your brain allows your stress level to get out of control, your immune system is suppressed. Well-managed stress, however, may help keep your immune system healthy. No one can completely avoid pressure in this world. What we can choose is a healthy balance.

Psychoneuroimmunology researchers have looked at many aspects of the body-mind connection, and each discovery seems to confirm that all of us can indeed become masters of our lives. The fruits of their approach are already being harvested in comprehensive programs of mind-body medicine at Harvard University, the University of Massachusetts, Stanford University, the University of Miami, and the University of California at San Francisco and Los Angeles. People with such life-threatening and debilitating illnesses as cancer, AIDS, coronary heart disease, and chronic pain are learning to change their habits and attitudes— what they eat, when they exercise, and how they think. A number of landmark studies have shown that these men and women are functioning far more effectively, feeling better, and, in some particularly striking instances, living longer.

Particularly impressive is the work of the late Dr. O. Carl Simonton, who made incredible advances with cancer patients using visualization. He reported that only about ten percent of the people who came to him were willing to do the work he recommended. The remainder would rather get the operation or the medication—anything to keep the reality "out there"—rather than look within and take charge.

There are those who receive a lot of value out of being victims. They can blame everybody else for their problems. They hold on to resentment and are unforgiving. Research has shown that many people have a difficult time processing emotions, and some evidence suggests that much of the sickness we experience comes, at least in part, from our inability to express anger, guilt, and fear. It is now well established that the repression of certain emotions can depress the body's ability to maintain a healthy immune function. Similarly, researchers are finding that our levels of stress and how we deal with them are main contributing factors to the state of our health.

For example, one of my clients, Steve, was on several project deadlines and was burning the candle at both ends for several weeks. He didn't have time to get much rest or relaxation. But his attitude was cheerful, he was always happy and saw the glass as half full. He had a passion for his work, and he knew that before too long he would have time to take a break and recuperate. His partner in the project, Richard, was working just as many hours but had a woe-is-me attitude; he bemoaned his fate, constantly complained about the long hours, and wished he worked somewhere else.

As the project deadlines came to an end, Steve felt invigorated and actually had energy to spare because he was able to deal with the stress. Richard, on the other hand, got the flu within a day of completing the work. It is fairly clear that his attitude helped drive up the levels of his stress hormones and suppressed his immune function. It was Abraham Lincoln who once said, "We are about as happy as we make up our minds to be." Steve chose to be happy. Richard suffered the consequences of both an out-of-balance life and a surly, negative attitude.

A whole-person approach that acknowledges the importance of stress and emotion is now seen by more and more professionals as the basis for recovery from all ailments and diseases. At its most basic, mental/behavioral therapy takes advantage of the mind-body connection and uses emotions to prod certain brain chemicals into stimulating the body's defense systems. Dr. Simonton's method of cancer treatment calls on the patient to alter feelings, attitudes, and expectations. Central to the process are daily exercises in relaxation and the use of imaging techniques, along with the physical activity necessary to reduce the stresses that he is convinced play a role in disease.

"If you get angry and that emotion doesn't get discharged, the resulting hormonal products and smaller particles such as neurotransmitters and endorphins don't get used," says Dr. Caroline Sperling, a clinical psychologist and director of the Cancer Counseling Institute in Bethesda, Maryland. "The residue remains and can become toxic in our bodies." The opposite is also true. "When you release those emotions effectively," she adds, "you get real well-being and adrenal charging so that the immune system stays strong and the body stays healthy."

According to Joan Borysenko, PhD, author of *Minding the Body, Mending the Mind* and co-founder and former director of the Mind/Body Clinic at New England Deaconess Hospital in Boston, messages conveying emotional reactions are transported instantaneously between the brain and a newly discovered site called a neuroreceptor on the white blood cells. So when someone is happy or thinks a joyful thought, the white blood cells, which are the body's primary defense system, receive that message immediately. Conversely, when someone's feelings are hurt, that message is transmitted directly to the white blood cells through the nervous system. All this happens very quickly, so that everything our minds react to is registered physically in our bodies. The discovery of the neuroreceptor site on the white blood cell is an exciting breakthrough.

Dr. Paul Rosch, president of the American Institute of Stress in New York, agrees that there is some very exciting work going on in psychoneuroimmunology, particularly in the area of visual imagery and cancer. "It has been determined that negative emotions have a high link to certain types of malignancies, and support for that comes from the observation that there are receptor sites on T-cell lymphocytes (a category of white blood cells) for certain brain chemicals, which suggests that there is a conversation going back and forth between the immune system and the brain," says Rosch.

Sperling concurs. "Imagery works like a computer to program into the hypothalamus the directions you want. It helps open up the parasympathetic nervous system so your body gets healthy. In other words, you're giving messages to your body, which translates them into neurotransmitters . . . to get the immune system to work better and the hormone system to calm down a little and stop creating abnormal cells."

Dr. Deepak Chopra gives what is perhaps the clearest explanation of all of the mind-body connection. He explains that the mind is in every cell of the body and that each thought causes a release of neuropeptides that are transmitted to all the cells in the body. Thoughts of Love, he says, causes the release of interleukin and interferon, which help heal the body. Anxious thoughts cause the release of cortisone and adrenaline, which suppress the immune system. Peaceful, calming thoughts release chemicals similar to Valium, which help the body to relax.

Norman Cousins, throughout his insightful book *Head First: The Biology of Hope*, presents evidence that hope, faith, Love, the will to live, purpose, laughter, and festivity help combat disease. Cousins writes, "The greatest force in the human body is the natural drive of the body to heal itself—but that force is not independent of the belief system, which can translate expectations into physiological change. Nothing is more wondrous about the 15 billion neurons in the human brain than their ability to convert thoughts, hopes, ideas, and attitudes into chemical substances. Everything begins, therefore, with belief. What we believe is the most powerful option of all."

The magnitude of impact that this inner belief system can have on healing is scientifically corroborated in the phenomenon known as the placebo effect. Medical researchers are well aware that a certain percentage of participants in medical studies who are treated with placebo drugs or procedures (treatments of no known medical value) will improve because they believe they have received a potent treatment. In the past, researchers tended to dismiss the placebo effect as a distraction, a confounding psychological variable that interfered with the real aims of the research. Yet the fact that belief can override the physiological insignificance of placebo medicines demonstrates the remarkable capability of this inner healing force.

While the messages from the brain through the nervous system are flashing instantaneously, another communication system is operating that is slower and steadier. Through our endocrine system, our thoughts trigger what's known as the hypothalamic-pituitary-adrenal axis, constantly bringing our bodies and emotions into alignment. Dr. Borysenko writes about studies on neuropeptides, a group of hormonal messengers (neurotransmitters) secreted by the brain, immune system, and digestive system. Endorphins, for example, which are commonly associated with the "runner's high" experienced by joggers, are among the several dozen neuropeptides researchers have identified. These substances represent a rich pharmacy of natural drugs that the body produces in response to various internal and external stresses.

Borysenko explains, "If you are fearful, for example, it is not just an emotion. It is that every cell in your body has now received a biochemical signal about fear broadcast by the neuropeptide system, and has changed its metabolism in some way." As exciting as these insights are, however, Borysenko adds an important caveat when she warns us not to exaggerate the connection between personality and disease. "It is not as if everyone who is hostile and cynical will have heart disease or that everyone who acts like a doormat will develop cancer," she explains. "Personality is only one of many variables that can affect health."

British cardiologist Dr. Peter Nixon explains that increased stress and arousal cause numerous changes in body functioning that eventually interfere with immune function, protein synthesis, and cardiac functioning. Repetitive stress also uses up the body's reserves, leading to increased stress on other physiological functions which, in turn, can result in heart disease, cancer, or depression.

A long time ago, Plato said that the physician who treats only the body and does not address the mind is not treating the whole patient. In 140 AD, the Roman physician Galen observed that it is depressed women who get breast cancer. The mind-body connection has always been evident to those prepared to see it; what is new is the growing body of scientific documentation that tells us how it works.

Clearly, this complex, dynamic interplay of attitudes, emotions, and physiology can be harnessed to promote our health and well-being—if we simply choose to make it work for us. How often have you felt your muscles tense when you were worried, or been recharged physically by a hug from a loved one? Emotional depression can translate into fatigue, and having fun with people we enjoy can create energy. It is within our power to take charge of our lives, thoughts, emotions, beliefs, and attitudes—to become the best we can be.

The lessons I've learned, and the many questions that have inspired me to think harder and clarify my own beliefs, have led me to emphasize balance as the key to a healthier, happier life. Here are some specific ways I've discovered, by distilling the messages of all the "Sacredness" chapters, to live in serenity and joy.

Make fitness and wellness the mainspring of everyday life.

Develop a well-rounded fitness program that includes strength training (weights), aerobics, and stretching or yoga. Make it a top priority. Nothing can do more to make you vibrantly healthy, energetic, and youthful than a regular fitness program. A study at Tufts University found that after one year of twice-a-week strength training, women's bodies were 16 to 20 years more youthful. The women in the study had less fat and more muscle, prevented or reversed bone loss, dramatically increased strength and energy, and showed surprising gains in balance and flexibility. No other program, including diet, medication, and aerobic exercise, has ever achieved comparable results. Learn more about this program in the book *Strong Women Stay Young*, by Miriam E. Nelson, PhD. Men, although they are generally more attuned to the benefits of strength training, should be aware of these results, too.

Make sure to get enough water and wholesome foods. Always try to eat your foods close to the way nature produced them. Get plenty of fresh air and healthy amounts of sunshine, too, and take saunas if you can, to help rid the body of toxins. Avoid dependence on caffeine, nicotine, alcohol, and drugs that interfere with your immune system's functioning. If you want to have a good influence on the health and fitness of those you love, take care of yourself. There is nothing stronger than the ripple effect of personal example. Not to mention that the only person's health and fitness you can change is your own. I love George Bernard Shaw's comment, "If you must hold yourself up to your children as an object lesson, hold yourself up as an example and not as a warning."

Get enough sleep.

According to a recent study by the National Sleep Foundation, even though 98 percent of us know that sleep is just as important to our health as nutrition and exercise, most adults fail to get sufficient sleep. Americans average seven and one-half hours of sleep a night. The ideal is ten. You read that right. Ten hours. In his excellent book, *Power Sleep*, Dr. James B. Maas claims that half the population of the United States is sleep-deprived. He also maintains that many Americans don't know what it's like to be fully alert and have become habituated to low levels of alertness. If you need an alarm clock to wake up, or if it's a struggle to get out of bed in the morning, or if you fall asleep in meetings or watching television, you are sleep-deprived.

Even minor sleep deprivation causes mood changes. People get angry and upset more easily, lose patience, and snap at one another. One of the first things to go when one is sleep-deprived is communication skills. Maas recommends taking 10- to 20-minute "power naps." Any longer than 20 minutes sends you into delta or deep sleep, and you wake up groggy. Also, if you nap too long in the afternoon, it will cause insomnia at night. Power naps pay back on the installment plan the debt we carry in our sleep-deficit banking account.

Never underestimate the importance of getting enough sleep. It is clearly an essential part of living a balanced life.

Learn to elicit a relaxation response.
With practice, anybody can become deeply relaxed in mind and body. Our nervous systems are bombarded every day by excessive environmental stimulation. Learn deep relaxation techniques such as meditation, yoga, and breathing exercises in order to keep stress levels under control. Every hour, take a deep breathing break instead of a coffee break. This simple action will do wonders to relieve stress, foster calmness, clear your mind, and help you to see your life from a higher, more positive perspective.

Be on guard against prolonged feelings of anger and depression.
Beware of unexpressed feelings, especially negative ones. People who do not express their feelings get sick more often, stay sick longer, and die sooner than expressive people. Non-expression of emotion and denial of hostility or anger are two of the factors most related to an unfavorable prognosis in cancer patients. Unexpressed negative feelings feed on themselves: anger, for instance, can turn against the Self and emerge as depression or severe anxiety. Negative emotions, as mentioned earlier, also trigger the release of substances that can suppress immune function.

Deal with problems in a way that lets you clear up your negative feelings as thoroughly and quickly as possible. Remember that feelings aren't good or bad, they just are. Sharing them with a trusted friend or other support person is healing.

Teach yourself to have positive expectations about everything in your life, including your wellness. There is a classic study of people about to have surgery. The first group of patients dreaded surgery and attempted to postpone or avoid it. The second group, with the same medical problems, regarded the surgery as an opportunity to rid themselves of their illnesses. After surgery, those who had had positive expectations had much better post-operative experiences. Such outcomes have been documented repeatedly.

The loss of a loved one tests our emotional balance severely. If a person is able to integrate loss into a broader texture and meaning of life, and feel grief and depression without losing the inner sense of safety, those feelings will be relatively temporary. But if someone responds to loss with prolonged depression, the body will also be in a state of depression, making that person susceptible and vulnerable to many ailments. When we can see ourselves as participants in life, rather than as victims of unfortunate circumstances, our lives automatically become less stressful and more wholesome.

Be aware of your thoughts.
What we think determines what we experience. Each of us has the freedom to accept and embrace whatever thoughts we choose. We possess within the silence of our being the ability to decide, create, and become whatever we want to become. Monitor what you're thinking and don't allow yourself to think negatively. Instead, think only about things you want to be part of your life.

Substitute forgiveness for judgment.
The strongest poison to the human spirit is the inability to forgive oneself or another person. The need to judge and control keeps you spiritually toxic. Choose to practice forgiveness and make no judgments. If you stop wanting to know why things happen as they do and instead let God guide your life, you reach a state of true serenity.

Feel the fear and let it go.
Fear is such a significant, powerful force that it always seems to come from outside ourselves. We feel it on many levels—physically, mentally, and emotionally. Often we don't begin the one thing we really want to do in life because of fear. Yet the greatest possible growth and personal development come from facing our pain and fear. I like what Jack Kornfield says in his wonderful book *A Path with Heart:* "The compartments we create to shield us from what we fear, ignore, and exclude exact their toll later in life. Periods of holiness and spiritual fervor can later alternate with opposite extremes—bingeing on food, sex, and other things—becoming a kind of spiritual bulimia. Spiritual practice

will not save us from suffering and confusion, it only allows us to understand that avoidance of pain does not help."

Recognize that your fears are just like other feelings—neither good nor bad. They just are, and all you risk by uncovering them is the amazing surprise that by acknowledging fear and moving on, you become healthier and more fully human.

Visualize your goals and dreams every day.
James Allen wrote these words 75 years ago, and they are just as true today: "You think in secret and it comes to pass. Environment is but your looking glass." He reminds us how creative we really are. Every day, spend a few minutes visualizing with your mind's eye not only your goals but also how you would like your life to be in every detail. In addition to visualizing, assume the feeling of the wish fulfilled.

Find time each day to be alone.
It is by spending time alone, breathing deeply, and quieting everyday thoughts that we can do the most for our happiness and peace of mind. Mother Teresa wrote, "We need to find God, and He cannot be found in noise and restlessness. God is the friend of silence." Silence nourishes the soul and heals the heart. Silence is always sacred, and solitude is necessary for deep silence. The word "alone" is derived from the Middle English phrase "all one." In solitude and silence, I see most clearly what is out of balance in my life, and in silence I feel the all-providing power that sustains me and is the Source of all creation. However brief it may be, find some time each day to enjoy the peace of your own company.

Practice some kind of meditation and prayer daily.

Meditation goes hand-in-hand with spending time alone each day. The physical benefits of meditation are as well documented as the mental and spiritual rewards. Research by Dr. Herbert Benson of Harvard University, author of *The Relaxation Response*, has shown that meditation not only improves immune function but is also associated with a host of positive physiological effects such as altered brain states, decreased heart rate, lower blood pressure, a relaxed body, and a more youthful appearance.

Too often we look outside ourselves for our worth, forgetting that nothing will ever be enough until we are enough. Meditating every day, listening to our inner guidance or intuition, reminds us that we are enough because we are not alone. Meditation nourishes faith and connects us to our Source, which I call God. Whether you call it meditation or prayer time, both reconnect you with the Divine. Each moment spent in peaceful prayer or meditation is like a coin put into a bank account. Choose to create a prosperous life rich with meditation/prayer time.

Simplify life.

Contrary to popular belief, we are not mere victims of our environment. When we yield to the pressure, we go faster and push harder without keeping life in perspective, growing more and more insensitive to our needs and the needs of those around us. It requires effort, but you can slow down. Discover the joy in simple pleasures.

- breathe deeply
- smell the flowers
- talk to the animals
- sing to the birds
- be with friends

- greet the sun
- seek out shooting stars
- scratch behind a kitty's ear
- make someone smile
- marvel at the miracle you are
- tell someone you love them
- laugh out loud and often

Nourish your sense of humor.

Yes, laughter is good for everybody. A bit of emotional detachment and hearty laughter every day really does stimulate the immune system. Humor aids most—and probably all—major systems of the body. A good laugh, Cousins said in one of his lectures I attended at UCLA, gives the heart muscles a healthy workout; improves circulation; fills the lungs with oxygen-rich air; clears the respiratory passages; acts on alertness hormones that stimulate various tissues; alters the brain by diminishing tension in the central nervous system; counteracts fear, anger, and depression, all of which are linked to physical illness; and helps relieve pain.

Laughter is the best demonstration that creating vibrant health can be fun. Try to move gracefully among all the activities of daily life without being ensnared by either outer demands or inner desires. Don't take life so seriously.

Slow down.

Early in the book I mentioned a recent *New York Times* article that claimed that one third of all Americans are always in a state of rushing. I suppose we don't need newspapers to tell us what's true. It's hard to celebrate ourselves and our lives or appreciate life's simple pleasures when we are always rushing around. Remember the passage I also mentioned from *The Little Prince* in which the prince is in the railway station watching all of the people rushing all over the place. When he asks someone where everyone is going, the person responds that even the engineer doesn't know where he's going. Well, that's a powerful statement—and no doubt truer today than it was 65 years ago when it was written. People are rushing all over the place and no one's sure where they're going.

How about you? Is your life one big rush after another? Do you wish you could slow down and be more present? Well, you can. And it's a choice you must make as you decide how best to create your great adventure—this amazing thing you call your life. In my favorite movie, *The Sound of Music*, the Captain says to the Baroness: "Activity suggests a life filled with purpose." In my private practice, people come to me all the time feeling totally stressed out because of all the things they need to do and all of the rushing around that's part of their daily experiences. On a plaque above my desk in my office, I have the following two simple reminders—"Let peace of mind be the organizing principle in your life" and "Let joy be your compass." I point this out to all of my stressed-out clients. When you choose to slow down, breathe more deeply, be aware of the present moment, and relish all of life's magical moments, you will bring more peace and joy into your body and life.

Nurture and develop your intuition.

Intuition is sometimes called a sixth sense, a hunch, a gut feeling, going on instinct, or just knowing deep inside. Psychologists consider it an obscure mental function that provides us with information, so that we know without knowing how we know. I believe intuition is the voice of God within each one of us. Intuition can be nurtured in a variety of ways that quiet the conscious mind—through meditating, gazing out a window, relaxing, or taking silent walks in nature. However you do it, the best way is to be still and listen. The more you trust and act on your intuitive hunches, the stronger and more readily available they become.

Be grateful.

The simple state of gratitude creates blessings. Be grateful for everything that's going on in your life, whatever the circumstances, for this attitude all by itself can foster happiness and peace of mind and assist you to live more fully. Remember that there is power in difficulty and challenge because they force us to tap reserves of courage, hope, faith, surrender, and Love we weren't aware we possessed.

We don't have to have problems in order to grow. We can grow in spiritual maturity every time we turn to God. Equally, it seems to me, faith in God and His goodness can give us the understanding and strength to be grateful in the midst of challenge. In *A Course in Miracles* it is said, "Love cannot be far behind a grateful heart and thankful mind. . . ." These are the true conditions for your homecoming."

When you live with gratitude, it is easy to bring happiness and reverence for life into your daily experiences. Greet each day with joy and enthusiasm regardless of circumstances, and be thankful for everything that touches you—the warm sun on your face, the food you eat, your family and friends, your surroundings, even the air you breathe. There is always something miraculous in life, even when we seem to have nothing. Take notice and enjoy the sacredness of every moment. Be grateful for the Divine in everyone and everything.

Encourage the child in you.

Young children seem to know how to make life a celebration and create magical moments. They see the everyday world as full of wonder and mystery, and with this perception, they infuse the most ordinary things with excitement. Children know how to open the door to the kingdom of wonder. Take their example: Don't plan your calendar down to the last minute. Be more flexible and leave time for spontaneity in daily activities. Practice forgiveness. Forget about being critical and judgmental. Let your inner child come out and play.

Live in the present.
Living in the moment is different from living for the moment. Children naturally live in the timelessness of the present, but we can learn to do it consciously. To be fully present each moment, we must free ourselves from the past, and the only way to achieve this freedom fully is to heal our past. If we don't, the past will repeat itself and keep us trapped in it. When we're trapped in the past, we're not here now; we can't be fully present and we can't pay attention to what's happening all around us. We must stop living our lives mechanically, unconsciously going over and over the same ground, and start paying attention to the present moment.

Don't spend time comparing the present with the past. Every new step you take is upon sacred ground. Every moment is imbued with wonder and miracles.

Give love and kindness.
At the most fundamental level, being loving and kind improves health. We all need love—and I'm not just talking about romantic attraction. That warm feeling we get from hugging a child, cheering a friend, being a good listener, or even treating ourselves to some little luxury boosts the immune system. Petting a dog or admiring fish in a tank lowers the blood pressure. In one study, people who watched a film of Mother Teresa tenderly caring for

sick children experienced the same heightened immune response as people who had recently fallen in love.

Whether we are at work or at play, with friends or with strangers, a friendly smile and a kind word can brighten someone's day and bring us rewards of health and happiness at the same time. Every day we also have opportunities to be kind and loving toward our environment by taking care of our home, planet Earth.

Act in caring, loving ways for your own sake and for the future sake of your children and all children everywhere. As Mother Teresa said, "Do ordinary things with extraordinary love." Led by Divine Guidance, welcome every opportunity to express love and kindness.

Live with integrity.

Make sure that who you appear to be is who you really are. Our inner realities—our beliefs, our commitments, our values—are all reflected on the outside in the way we live our lives from day to day. It takes a lot of energy to live without integrity, because it is emotionally and intellectually exhausting when the way we behave is not aligned with the way we are on the inside. Simply put, dishonesty is enervating.

Honesty and integrity go hand-in-hand. It was Thomas Jefferson who said, "Honesty is the first chapter in the book of wisdom." To be dishonest is to be partly forged, fake, or fictitious. To be honest is to be genuine, authentic, and real. Honesty is best cultivated by being honest; the more you choose honesty, the more it becomes a habit. The more you live with synchronicity in what you believe, think, feel, say, and do, the more peace and happiness you will invite into your life.

Develop high self-esteem and self-love.

High self-esteem is important for our own well-being and the well-being of everybody around us. If we have children, they learn from watching us live, and there is no more powerful influence on them. When we are living at our best, we are a positive model for everyone, so heal your emotional wounds of the past. Release your emotional baggage and treat yourself with the respect and kindness you deserve.

Of course we all have days when nothing seems to go right and we feel all bent out of shape like a weathered futtock on a sailing vessel. During these times, we must remind ourselves that life ebbs and flows. We have good days and not-so-good days, but our state of being always strives toward balance—toward our true and lovable nature. We just need to have enough confidence in ourselves to follow our inner guidance. To be true to ourselves is to be in a state of grace.

Be true to yourself by following your heart. To find out if you are being true to yourself, ask yourself these questions: If I weren't getting paid for what I'm doing, would I do it anyway? If I knew I had only one year to live, would I continue to do what I'm doing? If the answer is no, carefully consider how you can make different choices that will change your answer to yes. Self-love and self-esteem will shine in all the actions that come from the heart.

Your life is a reflection of how you feel about yourself. Oliver Goldsmith, the English poet, novelist, and dramatist, wrote, "You can preach a better sermon with your life than with your lips."

Live peacefully.

There can be no greater goal in life than peace. What asset could be of more value to us than unshakable calmness and tranquility?

What better evidence of spiritual strength could we have than a peaceful mind and heart?

Peace of mind comes from accepting what you can't control and taking responsibility for what you can. It grows out of faith in your higher power and your spiritual nature. It comes when you let go of guilt, fear, and doubt. It is the result of forgiving yourself and others for all human imperfections. When you forget the delusion that something, someday, will make you happy, you can concentrate on finding peace and contentment in the present moment. Inner peace is always in the here and now, waiting quietly for you to discover it.

Begin now.

I like to tell people in my workshops that the time you feel least like starting something is precisely the time to forge ahead. Just the physical act of beginning creates the momentum and energy that will allow you to travel beyond the fear and toward your greatest accomplishments. A healthy lifestyle is more than eating right and exercising regularly. Make a commitment to yourself to enrich each day physically, mentally, emotionally, and spiritually. By choosing to put this splendid balance into your life, you'll reap the rewards of living healthfully, vibrantly, and joyfully. Every step you take is on sacred ground. Everything about your life is sacred. The path to the sacred is your own body, heart, and mind; the history of your life; and all the closest relationships and circumstances that surround you. If not here, if not now, when and where can we engender joy, compassion, freedom, and happiness? Don't place any limitations on your dreams or your Creator by doubting that you can accomplish your soul's desire and live a sacred life.

You are not being called upon to change yourself. You are being asked to be more of what you already are. The invitation is bold, the stakes are high, and the outcome is certain. Dare to live your destiny now.
—ALAN COHEN

Courage is not the absence of fear but the triumph over it. Cast off your chains. Lead.
—NELSON MANDELA

The whole course of things go to teach us faith.
—RALPH WALDO EMERSON

If each of us would only sweep our own doorstep, the whole world would be clean.
—MOTHER TERESA

Appendix A

Workbook
Self-Discovery Questions and Action Choices

Take a deep breath and trust that life, despite its ups and downs,
is essentially wonderful.
—Thomas Kinkade

The whole of science is nothing more than a refinement
of everyday thinking.
—Albert Einstein

The following questions and suggestions are designed to support
you in learning more about yourself and in creating your own
personal pathway to vibrant health. Space is provided to write
your responses in the book, but if you find it isn't enough, please
don't hesitate to use extra paper.

In the search to "know thyself," there aren't any right or
wrong answers. As you deepen your self-discovery, the workbook
will allow you to refer back to earlier ideas and add new ones.
It will be there to help and encourage you as you make positive
changes in your attitudes, thoughts, beliefs, actions, and lifestyle.
The Self-Discovery Questions and Action Choices are grouped to
emphasize specific themes in the book. Don't skip over this part!

HOW WILL I CELEBRATE MYSELF?
Self-Discovery Questions

1. What does it mean to me to be healthy? How would I feel if I were in perfect
   health?

2. Have I received value from being unwell in the past? Would someone pay more attention to me, for example?

3. In the past, whom have I blamed, or what situations have I blamed, for my failures?

4. How do people treat me? Assuming that I've taught them how to treat me by the way I treat myself, what changes can I make in myself and my behavior that will support my newfound magnificence?

5. Have I ever felt limited in what I could be or do because of what others have said about me? As I let go of limiting opinions and beliefs and tune in to my own inner signals, what new possibilities become exciting and available to me?

Action Choices

1. Following is a list of at least five things I love about myself:

2. These are a few things I can do to increase my self-confidence and self-image:

3. Because I must take myself with me everywhere I go, I now choose to start loving myself unconditionally and consistently. Following is a description of myself as the radiant being I am:

4. Here are some of the reasons why I deserve to be optimally healthy and fully functioning:

5. I choose to find myself more attractive than ever before. I am wonderful. I now take a few minutes to paint a word picture of myself as the exquisite person I am, emphasizing my many positive qualities:

HOW WILL I EMBRACE MY AUTHENTIC SELF?
Self-Discovery Questions

1. What do I feel angry about?

2. What do I feel upset about?

3. What do I feel depressed or hopeless about?

4. What things have caused me anxiety in the past?

5. What am I feeling happy and joyful about?

6. What specific time can I set aside each day to be by myself and relax?

7. What people in my life can I ask for help in eliminating negative thoughts and words?

Action Choices

1. I will sit quietly with my eyes closed for the next few minutes, envisioning myself as a peaceful, relaxed, confident, and happy person. Then I will describe exactly how that looked and felt:

2. Before I go to sleep at night, I will sit quietly and forgive myself and anyone else I feel has hurt me in any way. These are the people who need my immediate attention:

3. I will choose one person with whom I have not been feeling in harmony, close my eyes, and picture us facing each other in a circle of white or pink light. I will lovingly share my feelings with that person and resolve any conflict, then finish by seeing our hearts connect in unconditional love. I will describe my ideal relationship with this person:

4. If I need to forgive a person who has passed away, I will sit down and write that individual a letter offering forgiveness and love. These are the feelings I will express:

5. If I know someone who is experiencing lots of stress, anxiety, depression, hopelessness, or helplessness, I will contact that person as soon as possible and encourage him or her to talk while I listen without judging, criticizing, or offering advice. This is someone I know who needs a friend simply to listen and care:

6. From this day forward, I will give this many hugs a day:

7. I know now that the better I handle stress, the healthier and happier I'll be. Here are some ways I've handled stress in the past:
   This is how I choose to deal with stress from now on, in ways that support my immune system and well being:

HOW WILL I LIVE MY HIGHEST VISION?
Self-Discovery Questions

1. Am I living my ideal life now? If not, why not?

2. What are my goals in the following areas?
   Relationships
   Career
   Finances
   Fitness
   Interests and Hobbies

Health

Spirituality

3. If I knew I couldn't fail, what would I do in my life?

Action Choices

1. Following is my ideal vision of myself, living my ideal life. This is how my life would be, how the world around me would be, and how I would feel:

2. These are changes I can make immediately that will move me closer to my vision:

3. Listed below are the words and phrases that I now choose to eliminate from my vocabulary:

4. In order to create relationships the way I want them to be, I will not try to change anyone else but will change my own thoughts and attitudes in the following ways:

HOW WILL I CHOOSE TO BE HEALTHY?

Self-Discovery Questions

1. What foods do I need to eliminate from my diet because they don't support my health?

2. In what ways have I been treating myself without love through my eating behaviors?

3. How can I change the way I prepare food in order to increase my health and well-being?

4. What beliefs do I hold about food that sabotage my healthiness?

Action Choices

1. Benjamin Franklin informed the world that whatever we can do for 21 days becomes a habit. For 21 days I will eliminate the following from my diet and add the following to my diet:

2. Starting today with the first thing on the list, I will use these books, magazines, or tapes to assist me in my health program:

3. Listed here are some supplements that I now choose to include in my nutritional program to enhance my health:

4. Following are at least five affirmations that support my being vibrantly healthy:

5. Each day I will spend at least ten minutes visualizing myself as a healthy, radiant being who treats herself or himself respectfully and lovingly. This is precisely how I will appear in my vision:

HOW WILL I GET FIT FOR LIFE?
Self-Discovery Questions
1. How do I feel about exercise?
2. Which fitness activities do I, or can I, engage in that I enjoy?
3. What beliefs do I have about my body that have been working against me?
4. What excuses seem to come up frequently that interfere with my exercising?

Action Choices
1. Here are my exercise and fitness goals for the following month, three months, six months, and year:
2. The areas of my body that need special attention, and the exercises that will address them, are:
3. My body, whatever its level of fitness, is splendiferous. Here are a few of the miraculous things it can do, for which I am grateful:
4. The supremely fit Self I visualize while I am working out looks like this:

HOW WILL I LET MY HEART-LIGHT SHINE?
Self-Discovery Questions
1. In what areas of my life am I too serious?
2. Would I describe myself as a happy, positive person? Am I the type of person I would like to have for a friend?
3. How do I feel when I am around children?
4. What qualities do I see in children that I'd like to integrate more fully into my own life?
5. In what areas of my life am I too rigid and orderly—too "adult"?
6. How often do I give myself permission to act silly and crazy?
7. Do I spend my present moments feeling guilty about the past or worrying about the future, or do I truly embrace the here and now?

Action Choices

1. If I were to let the child in me out to explore, play, and be spontaneous and creative, my life would change in the following ways:

2. In order to get more in touch with my inner child, I am going to spend some time observing children at play, as well as participating with them. I can do this in the following ways:

3. These are some fun things I can do for those I care about (for example, write a special note, send flowers, or record a song):

4. Here are some things I tried in the past six months that I had never tried before:

5. Here are some new ventures I choose to undertake in the coming six months:

6. Here are some changes I can make to lighten up and become a little less serious:

7. I will choose one of the following people I have wanted to meet or know better and make plans to get together next week:

8. Now that I spend time visualizing my ideal life every day, I will take the next few moments to imagine one of my goals as already achieved. This is how I feel:

HOW WILL I EMBRACE THE SACRED WITHIN AND AROUND ME?
Self-Discovery Questions

1. What do I want most out of life?

2. What is my personal definition of success?

3. What does peace mean to me, and when do I feel most happy and at peace?

4. How do I feel about being alone?

5. What are things I do to avoid being alone and having quietude?

6. How old do I feel?

7. What past changes in my attitude have enriched my life?

8. If I knew I had just one year to live, what changes would I make now? What has kept me from making them already?

Action Choices

1. These are some ways I will spend the time during each day that I have set aside just for me:

2. Following are ways I choose to simplify my life:

3. In the past, my negative emotions have sometimes immobilized me. This is ending, because I will now take action and show my mettle instead, in the following ways:

4. If this were the last year of my life, the following things would be most important to me:

5. These are some changes I can make in my life to experience more peace:

6. Here is a list of affirmations that support my power to share peacefulness and enrich life on this planet:

There is a time for everything, and a season for every activity under heaven.
—ECCLESIASTICS 3:1

These are only hints and guesses,
Hints followed by guesses, and the rest
Is prayer, observance, discipline, thought and action.
—T.S. ELIOT

The lowest ebb is the turn of the tide.
—LONGFELLOW

Affirmations for Sacred, Balanced Living

A longing fulfilled is sweet to the soul.
—PROVERBS 13:19

There are only two ways to live your life. One is as though nothing is a miracle. The other is as though everything is a miracle.
—ALBERT EINSTEIN

Here is a sampling of one hundred affirmations, divided into four categories: Health, Prosperity, Spirituality, and Self-Esteem & Lifestyle. Use any or all of them as is, or change them to fit your own desires and goals, adding new ones to the list as you go. Consider writing your favorites on small cards to place in your home or office so you can see and use them often. When you say, write, or think an affirmation, you are "acting as if." Choose affirmations you can repeat until you feel them as true. At that point they become a part of your subconscious self-definition.

HEALTH

1. I am grateful for nature's abundance of delicious, nutritious foods.
2. I am the picture of health; I radiate verve and vitality.
3. My body is healing and rejuvenating itself moment by moment.
4. I live in harmony with nature and provide my body with the best of everything.
5. I give thanks for increasing health, fitness, prosperity, and love.
6. My sleep is relaxing, rejuvenating, and refreshing.

7. My body is an expression of my love for life, a miracle of youthfulness.
8. Raw foods are my favorite foods and I emphasize them in my daily diet.
9. My body is God's gift to me and what I am becoming is my gift to God.
10. I take time each day to relax, turn within, breathe deeply, and let go of tension.
11. Exercise is a top priority in my life and I find ways to be active daily.
12. I manage the stress in my life the same way I walk—with ease and grace.
13. My food choices reflect my love for myself and life.
14. I enjoy colorful, plant-based foods and choose to eat a variety each day.
15. I am losing weight and feeling great.
16. I take responsibility for my wellness lifestyle.
17. I have all the energy I need to accomplish my goals and fulfill my desires.
18. Today I renew my commitment to being healthy and resolve to make my word count.
19. I have an abundance of energy and my body is free of aches and pains.
20. I eat foods that nourish my body and mind and boost my self-esteem.
21. I fall asleep at night effortlessly and wake up feeling refreshed.
22. I love my body and treat it like royalty.
23. My healthy, active lifestyle brings me great joy and appreciation for life.
24. Day by day, I am becoming healthier and more confident about all of my choices.
25. I love to work out and I do so each and every day.
26. Vibrant health is my natural state of being.
27. I breathe in health and vitality and exhale all tensions and worries.

PROSPERITY

28. I am worthy of receiving the unlimited offerings of the universe.
29. I always prosper in everything I do.
30. The more I give in love, the more I am given.
31. Everywhere I look I see opportunities to prosper.
32. An avalanche of abundance is flowing to me now.
33. I accept and expect prosperity in every area of my life.
34. I am attracting the people, circumstances, and resources to make my dreams come true.

35. The more I trust my intuition, the more prosperity comes my way.

36. I am amply rewarded for my creative ideas.

37. I rejoice in my continuing good fortune.

38. I am the creator of my life, and I choose to create a passionate adventure filled with success.

SPIRITUALITY

39. My will and Divine Will are one.

40. I release all my fear and worry and trust that all things are working together for my highest good.

41. I love to be outdoors to celebrate the spectacular beauty in nature.

42. A loving, powerful spirit moves through me, lighting my path.

43. I trust myself and my intuitive nature.

44. I give thanks and praise for all things and choose to be radiantly happy.

45. I welcome Spirit's guidance with an open, grateful mind and heart.

46. With each breath I take, I center my thoughts on being loving and peaceful.

47. My life is a harmonious expression of the insights and values of my higher self.

48. Each morning I give thanks for the gift of life and the beauty all around me.

49. In quiet and solitude I listen to the whisperings of Divine Inspiration in me.

50. Divine healing energy is flowing through me now, cleansing, purifying and renewing every cell in my body.

51. I surrender to life and behold the Divine in everyone and everything.

SELF-ESTEEM & LIFESTYLE

52. I release my fears and insecurities and replace them with faith and confidence.

53. Everything about my life is sacred to me.

54. I am committed to living my highest potential in every area of my life.

55. I celebrate life today and every day.

56. All my goals and desires are coming to fruition in my life now.

57. I am the master of my life and I have the power to create anything I desire.

58. I greet each day with a thankful and cheerful heart.

59. I love and value myself very much.

60. I communicate my feelings openly, lovingly, and honestly with my partner, family, friends, and coworkers.
61. I deserve to be happy, live fully, and celebrate life.
62. My home is my sanctuary and is filled with love, peace, and joy.
63. I receive great pleasure in pleasing my partner and do so often.
64. I am true to myself.
65. I am grateful for all life's lessons that bless me richly.
66. I live in a peaceful world, because I am a peaceful person.
67. I appreciate the people in my life and tell them, in special ways, what they mean to me.
68. I embrace each day with enthusiasm and find ways to uplift others.
69. I seek out new adventures and move out of my comfort zone.
70. I find ways to express my feelings of hurt in honest, loving ways.
71. All things are working together for good in my life, and I trust in the process.
72. I choose to surround myself with beauty and positive people.
73. I always treat others the way I would like to be treated—with kindness and respect.
74. I see all challenges as positive opportunities.
75. All that my heart desires is coming into my life now.
76. I live simply and pay attention to what's really essential.
77. I am grateful for all opportunities to grow and transform.
78. I am lovable, confident, and self-assured.
79. I draw to myself positive people who share my zest for life.
80. I take responsibility for my life, release blame, and let go of what no longer serves my highest good.
81. Today I find ways to simplify my life and all my affairs.
82. Today and every day I let my inner child come out to play and celebrate life.
83. I am luminescent and I choose to live each day with vigor, vim, and valor. (Or keep adding "v's"—veracity, vitality, vivacity, verve!)
84. I release the past and embrace each moment with love.
85. I find ways to show my appreciation for myself and others.
86. Because I respect myself and others, I arrive on time and keep my word.
87. My body is sexy and beautiful.
88. I let the tranquility that's in my heart infuse my intentions.

89. My persistence and determination work miracles.
90. I love myself unconditionally.
91. I am at peace with myself and the universe.
92. I make a positive difference in the world and have an impact on those around me.
93. I give thanks for every experience that I have.
94. My old pains no longer hurt me. They have become a distant memory.
95. I embrace change, knowing that it transforms my life.
96. I give thanks for my new life and my new motivation to be the best I can be.
97. I bless and forgive everyone who has caused me pain; I let go of the past; I am free.
98. I choose to experience peace of mind.
99. Today I make a fresh start and begin to live on higher ground.
100. I have a clear vision of what I want to achieve and I see it happening now.

The first wealth is health.
—RALPH WALDO EMERSON

Be still and discover your center of peace.
—TAO

I am certain of nothing but of the holiness of the heart's affections and the truth of imagination.
—JOHN KEATS

Live in each season as it passes; breathe air, drink the drink, taste the fruit, and resign yourself to the influences of each. Let them be your only diet drink and botanical medicines.
—HENRY DAVID THOREAU

About the Author

The more you love, and the more you're loved,
the lovelier you are.
—June B. Smith (Susan's mom)

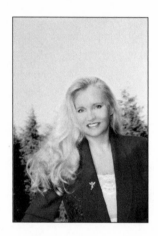

For a woman with three of America's most ordinary names, Susan Smith Jones, MS, PhD, certainly has made extraordinary contributions in the fields of optimum holistic health, fitness, nutrition, longevity, and human potential. Selected as one of ten "Healthy American Fitness Leaders" by the President's Council on Physical Fitness & Sports, Susan is an award-winning writer and advice columnist. She has authored over 1,500 magazine articles, numerous audio programs, and 25 books. Susan appears regularly in the pages and on the covers of national and international publications and has been a guest on more than 2,000 radio and television talk shows around the country and worldwide. For 30 years, she taught students, staff, and faculty at UCLA how to be healthy and fit. On her frequent lecture and media tours, she discusses how to look younger and live longer; boost immunity and energy; maximize wellness in the workplace; enhance management training and conflict resolution; minimize stress and maximize joy; prevent and alleviate disease; use food as medicine; set up a healthful kitchen; create meals that rejuvenate the body; detoxify the body with whole foods and fresh juices; make tasty blender meals in seconds; raise healthy children; and bring a sacred balance into your body and life.

An acclaimed holistic health and lifestyle coach, private culinary instructor, and natural foods chef, Susan works with discerning clients around the world. She creates menus and rejuvenation programs designed to support and complement the needs of her individual clients, as well as the participants at her specialized holistic health retreats. In addition, she serves as a recipe developer and product consultant for the health industry.

Susan's inspiring messages and innovative techniques for achieving total health in body, mind, and spirit have won her a grateful and enthusiastic following and have put her in constant demand internationally as a health and fitness consultant and motivational speaker for community, corporate, and religious or spiritual groups. She also is president of Health Unlimited, a consulting firm dedicated to the advancement of health education, corporate efficacy and wellness, and peaceful, balanced living that she founded in Los Angeles and now operates in both the United States and the United Kingdom.

Many years ago, when a devastating car accident fractured Susan's back so severely that doctors told her she would never again be physically active and would live a life of chronic pain, she proved them wrong. Her miraculous recovery proved to her that we all have within ourselves everything we need to live our lives to the fullest. She now regularly participates in a variety of fitness activities, including hiking, weight training, in-line skating, biking, Pilates, horseback riding, and yoga. A gifted teacher, Susan brings together modern research and ageless wisdom in all of her work. She resides in West Los Angeles.

www.SusanSmithJones.com

If you can make one heap of all your winnings
And risk it on one turn of pitch-and-toss,
And lose, and start again at your beginnings
And never breathe a word about your loss;
If you can force your heart and nerve and sinew
To serve your turn long after they are gone,
And so hold on when there is nothing in you
Except the Will which says to them: "Hold on";

If you can talk with crowds and keep your virtue,
Or walk with kings—nor lose the common touch;
If neither foes nor loving friends can hurt you;
If all men count with you, but none too much;
If you can fill the unforgiving minute
With sixty seconds' worth of distances run -
Yours is the Earth and everything that's in it,
And—which is more—you'll be a Man my son!
—Rudyard Kipling

To Our Readers

Conari Press, an imprint of Red Wheel/Weiser, publishes books on topics ranging from spirituality, personal growth, and relationships to women's issues, parenting, and social issues. Our mission is to publish quality books that will make a difference in people's lives--how we feel about ourselves and how we relate to one another. We value integrity, compassion, and receptivity, both in the books we publish and in the way we do business.

Our readers are our most important resources, and we value your input, suggestions, and ideas about what you would like to see published. Please feel free to contact us, to request our latest book catalog, or to be added to our mailing list.

Conari Press
An imprint of Red Wheel/Weiser, LLC
500 Third Street, Suite 230
San Francisco, CA 94107
www.redwheelweiser.com